C000178756

PHYSIQUE SECRETS

PHYSIQUE SECRETS

The Complete Playbook for Building

an Amazing Male Body

NICK SCHLAGER

© Copyright 2022 - All rights reserved.

It is not legal to reproduce, duplicate, or transmit any part of this document either by electronic means or in printed format. Recording of this publication is strictly prohibited, and any storage of this document is not allowed unless with written permission from the publisher, except for the use of brief quotations in a book review.

Disclaimer: Please note that the information contained within this document is for educational and entertainment purposes only. All effort has been executed to present accurate, up-to-date, reliable, complete information. No warranties of any kind are declared or implied. Readers acknowledge that the author is not engaged in the rendering of legal, financial, medical, or professional advice. The content within this book has been derived from various sources. Please consult a licensed professional before attempting any techniques outlined in this book.

Cover Design - Morgane Leoni
Book Formatting - Morgane Leoni
Illustrator - Sophia Lappe (www.sophialappe.com, contact@sophialappe.com)

MUSCLE IS STRONG, AND KNOWLEDGE IS POWERFUL.

BUT BOTH ARE USELESS WITHOUT CONSISTENT IMPROVEMENT

AND PRACTICAL APPLICATION.

TABLE OF CONTENTS

Introduction   9

Chapter 1: **Why You Should Read Physique Secrets**   12

Part I: The Strategy   16

SECRET 1 - HOW TO CONSTRUCT AN AMAZING PHYSIQUE

Chapter 2: **The Blueprint for Aesthetics**   18

Chapter 3: **The Power of Strength Training**   24

Chapter 4: **The Power of Flexible Dieting**   28

Part II: The Science   32

SECRET 2 - THE SIMPLE SCIENCE OF DEVELOPING MUSCLE AND STRENGTH

Chapter 5: **The Four Pillars of Building Muscle**   34

Chapter 6: **The Most Common Muscle-Building Mistakes Men Keep Making**   46

SECRET 3 - THE SIMPLE SCIENCE OF GETTING LEAN

Chapter 7: **The Four Pillars of Weight Change**   56

Chapter 8: **The Most Common Mistakes and Misconceptions That Halt Men's Fat Loss** 69

Part III: The Program Variables   78

SECRET 4 - EVERYTHING YOU NEED TO CREATE AN EFFECTIVE NUTRITION PROGRAM

Chapter 9: **Your Only Four Guidelines for Effective Dieting**   80

Chapter 10: **How Much to Eat for the Perfect Cut or Bulk**   84

Chapter 11: **Macronutrients for Optimal Muscle Growth and Fat Loss**   91

Chapter 12: **What to Eat for Optimal Health and Satiety**   96

Chapter 13: **The Truth about Nutrient Timing for Accelerating Your Results**   103

Chapter 14: **How to Schedule Your Meals and Nutrients to Put Your Life on Autopilot** 107

SECRET 5 – HOW TO TRAIN TO TRANSFORM YOUR PHYSIQUE QUICKLY

Chapter 15: **Turning Simple Science Into Optimized Training Variables**   113
Chapter 16: **The Three Most Important Training Variables**   115
Chapter 17: **How to Consistently Build More Muscle and Strength**   122

SECRET 6 – YOUR TRAINABLE MUSCLES, WHAT THEY DO, AND THE BEST EXERCISES FOR DEVELOPING THEM

Chapter 18: **Selecting the Best Strength-Training Exercises**   131
Chapter 19: **The Five Key Exercises for All-Around Muscle**   134
Chapter 20: **Your Muscles and How to Train Them**   144

Part IV: The Routine   162

SECRET 7 – SETTING THE STAGE FOR CONTINUOUS IMPROVEMENTS

Chapter 21: **Laying the Groundwork for Accelerated Results**   164
Chapter 22: **The Power of Routine**   166
Chapter 23: **The Correct Ways to Track and Measure Body Changes**   172

Part V: The Application   178

SECRET 8 – DESIGNING A TRAINING PROGRAM FOR BUILDING AN AMAZING BODY

Chapter 24: **How to Implement the Training Program Variables**   180
Chapter 25: *Physique Secrets* **Strength-Training Programs**   185
Chapter 26: **Implementing Exercise Manipulation**   202

SECRET 9 – CREATING A BODY-TRANSFORMING NUTRITION PROGRAM

Chapter 27: **Introduction to Meal Plan Construction**   208
Chapter 28: **Your Targets for Flexible Dieting Success**   210

Chapter 29: **How to Easily Create a Meal Plan Step-by-Step from Scratch**   215

Chapter 30: **How to Get Started Correctly**   232

Part VI: The Progression   238

SECRET 10 – HOW TO CONSISTENTLY GET THE BEST POSSIBLE RESULTS

Chapter 31: **Starting Your Body-Recomposition Momentum**   240

Chapter 32: **Optimizing Your Training Program for Consistent Strength and Muscle Gains**   245

Chapter 33: **How to Get a Lifetime of Consistent Results from Your Diet**   250

SECRET 11 – TIPPING THE SCALES

Chapter 34: **The Small Things That Can Help Give a Final Push**   255

Chapter 35: **Cardio for Aesthetics**   259

Chapter 36: **The Few Supplements Worth Adding to Your Regimen**   263

The Conclusion: **The End Is Just the Beginning**   269

Help Me Help You Better   271

References   272

INTRODUCTION

Thousands of normal men transform their bodies every single day. They improve their health, increase their muscle mass and strength, and easily lose unwanted body fat.

Yet the vast majority of men will fail.

Most men will struggle day in and day out just to make the scale budge or to put on a single pound of muscle.

They will consistently work out and diet, yet still be stuck for months, maybe even years, while never knowing exactly how to get the results they want, let alone keep them.

I've been there. I know how frustrating it can be to keep pushing yourself and working out without seeing improvement. I understand the struggle of trying to do everything correctly, only to fail yet again.

Like many men, I was not blessed with golden muscle-building genetics. So I had to work hard in the gym—but I worked even harder poring over the books and research to finally get to where I am now.

I wasted time, money, and energy that I will never get back. I spent years trapped in an endless cycle of superhard work and strict dieting just to pack on a couple of pounds of muscle over a period of months, only to watch it fade away in a quarter of the time.

Those years of failure led to years of taking the most respected training courses; reading the top-rated, overly scientific books; attending seminars; training with professional bodybuilders; and being trained by collegiate strength and conditioning coaches.

I don't want anyone else to go through the physical and emotional struggles I went through, so I took everything I know, condensed it to only what you actually need to know to get results, and put it into this book.

So, if you're looking for a complete playbook for any man to follow to build the ultimate male body, then you're in the right place.

Physique Secrets has been years in the making, but the primary goals have always remained the same:

1. To give you "literarily" everything you need—nothing more, nothing less—to build an amazing male physique.

2. To provide the most up-to-date science and research behind optimizing your muscle growth, strength, fat loss, health, and aesthetics.

3. To present everything in an easy-to-understand, "do this, don't do that" format so anyone can achieve results as efficiently as possible for the rest of his life.

These three goals make *Physique Secrets* the last (and only) muscle-building, fat-loss, strength-training, and nutrition book you will need to build an aesthetic physique.

Despite all the turmoil you may have gone through, you can still sculpt a truly fantastic body, both inside and out, no matter the circumstances. And in *Physique Secrets*, I will show you how.

Just as the book title suggests, I am here to reveal the secrets. You'll discover the truth behind how to eat and train like the hard-to-find and expensive fitness and nutrition experts so that you can get consistently better results as efficiently as possible.

You see, over the past 50 years, the science and research on building an amazing male physique have evolved exponentially. What used to be a lot of guesswork and relying on feelings by old-school bodybuilders, professional athletes, everyday gym-goers, and strength and conditioning coaches has become increasingly precise.

Since the early 2000s and even within the last few years, many new, high-quality research studies and meta-analyses have come incredibly close to proving the best ways to eat and train to optimize a man's results.

Unfortunately, the truth is hidden behind a trove of misinformation and even blatant lies.

So, to start, I want to let you in on a few secrets. Secrets that experts know to be true because hundreds of research studies have proven them time and time again.

First, any man can build an incredible body, inside and out, by building muscles, becoming impressively strong, leaning out, and improving his health and well-being.

Second, you can build an incredible physique no matter your genetics, current body type, goals, available time, food preferences, lifestyle, what you've tried in the past, etc. Whether you're tall, short, skinny, fat, big, or small, you have the power to drastically transform your body.

Third, it isn't as complicated or as difficult as many men are led to believe. In fact:

- You don't have to live in the gym to build a fantastic body.

- You don't have to train superhard until you are completely drained, sore, and struggling to breathe.

- You don't need to spend hours on a treadmill or stair stepper daily to be lean.

- You don't need to buy the latest gimmick or fancy workout equipment sold by some Instagram influencer to fast-track your transformation.

- You don't have to follow a fad diet or any special eating schedule to lose weight and stay fit.

- You don't need to stick to salads and "rabbit food" all your life to be healthy.

- You don't need to deny yourself your favorite foods or obsess over "clean eating" to shed body fat.

- You can get worse results by following old-school bodybuilders' advice.

- You don't need to spend hundreds of dollars a month on supplements hawked by steroid-fueled bodybuilders to gain strong and aesthetic muscles.

Unfortunately, these myths are just scratching the surface. There are many more things that steer so many people away from achieving real, noticeable, and rapid results.

That's why I created *Physique Secrets*: to debunk these myths and give you the facts—the secrets to acquiring your dream physique that the industry doesn't want you to know.

So, *Physique Secrets* is for you if you want to pack on muscle, get incredibly strong, drop down to a low-double-digit or even a single-digit body fat percentage, vastly improve your health, and learn the secrets experts use to get rapid results with less effort—the secrets most gym-goers don't even know they don't know.

It's time to stop being among the vast majority of men who struggle and fail in their body transformation journeys.

Physique Secrets can guide you on your journey. All you need to do is take that first step by flipping to the next section.

CHAPTER 1

WHY YOU SHOULD READ PHYSIQUE SECRETS

I signed up for my first strength and conditioning course about 10 years ago. I had been lifting weights for about 6 years and was an NCAA Division I athlete. I read a lot of bodybuilding articles online and watched YouTube videos from popular fitness coaches each week, and I thought I knew what I was doing.

It took about a week into the course to realize I knew next to nothing about strength training and nutrition.

I spent the rest of the course unlearning what I had previously thought and trying to figure out how to apply the proven science and research.

It was as though the first 6 years of my journey had been a waste of time. Sure, it can all be counted as a learning experience, but it was a long and expensive learning experience that I could have easily avoided.

That single class provided a significant course correction. It launched my long journey of delving into the science and research behind everything fitness and nutrition, especially when it came to building amazing bodies visually and functionally.

Over the next 3 to 4 years, I spent thousands of hours learning all about the science of fitness and nutrition.

I knew the vocabulary, the physiology of muscles, the biochemistry of nutrients and energy, human anatomy and kinesiology, how to time my nutrients to stay anabolic the whole day, the best exercises for targeting every single muscle, the advanced training techniques to trigger optimal muscle growth, and more.

Yet there still wasn't much change in the mirror, on the scale, or in the weight room. I had spent all this time studying but still failed the actual test.

I ran into the same problem many men face, regardless of experience and knowledge. I couldn't turn market content and scientific information into actionable steps for real-world results. I didn't have a system in place to take me from my current body and guide me step-by-step to an amazing physique.

THE POWER OF A SYSTEMATIC APPROACH TO BUILDING AN AMAZING PHYSIQUE

A system is a repeatable process for achieving a specific result. Systems are designed to ensure efficiency, minimize failures, provide proper progression, eliminate variables that don't matter, reduce confusion and wasted effort, and allow for continual improvement and success.

You can find systems being used in Fortune 500 companies, governments, computer programming, cars, your body, and even people's daily routines.

After years of learning, training, failing, and coaching others, I realized that building a muscular, strong, and lean body requires more than just in-depth knowledge, a meal plan, or a workout plan.

The people who get the best results and have the best bodies follow a series of steps, whether they're aware of them or not. They might not be efficient at moving from step to step and might fail every now and then, but they eventually hit each step.

By the end, they have a complete understanding of what they need to do, how to do it, and how to keep getting results for life without yo-yoing and confusion.

When I decided to write *Physique Secrets*, I didn't want to provide a lot of information but leave you confused about what to do with that information. I wanted to clarify the processes needed to build muscle, strength, and aesthetics based on what works in the real world, and on the most up-to-date research. Then, once I'd defined a clear process, I could systemize the steps.

By systemizing the process and its steps, you can see how everything works individually and together, how your diet and training affect each other, how the different variables that make up dieting and training affect the whole program, and how to consistently improve your training, your diet, your body, and your life.

This might seem overwhelming and like a lot of work, but by following a systematic approach rather than just walking into the gym or kitchen with a plan on a piece of paper, you can run your training, dieting, and life on autopilot.

Instead of focusing all your efforts on every little detail or worrying about whether you're doing things correctly, you'll be free to focus on consistently improving the systems to get better results with less effort.

We are all busy, so learning how to implement a body transformation system and then actually implementing it might feel like extra work. But in actuality, this systematic approach will make your life easier.

After all, that's the point of systems: to get repeatable results while minimizing failure, extra effort, and wasted time.

THE *PHYSIQUE SECRETS* SYSTEM

The *Physique Secrets* system isn't some workout program or diet regimen designed to sound fancy and sell a lot of books. It's not a social media challenge that you do for 90 days and then go about your life once finished.

It's the steps you should take and the order of events you need to follow to get results efficiently and for the rest of your life.

It's a system of practical knowledge and real-world implementation to help you create the strongest foundation for building an incredible physique.

This sounds more complicated than it is. But it will make more sense once you see the process and how everything flows together.

The large-scale system has only six parts. Inside each part, there are smaller systems to split topics and concepts into easier-to-understand but often misunderstood "secrets."

The secrets are detailed in the book's chapters, which will give you each step of the process of sculpting your desired physique.

Here are the six parts of the *Physique Secrets* system:

1. **The Strategy:** We start *Physique Secrets* by outlining an end goal and a strategy to get there. To get results in any endeavor, you must first know what it means to get results. Once you know what you're trying to achieve, you can determine the best tools for the job and a strategy for using them.

2. **The Science:** You can't improve your body if you don't know how it works. But trying to learn everything is a waste of time and effort. By homing in on what you need to know (and only what you need to know) about the science of building muscles, increasing strength, and leaning out, you can learn enough to get specific results without fluff or overwhelm.

3. **The Program Variables:** Once you understand how your body works, you can transition to understanding how the science applies to variables you can put into practice. Both strength training and dieting have many variables that will directly impact whether or not someone will see results, and the type of results a person can achieve. These variables combine to create a complete program in which one variable relies on the others. We will cover the optimal program variables so you know what to put into practice and, more importantly, what to avoid.

4. **The Routine:** You won't know if you're getting quality results from your system if you don't track and measure the outputs. You also can't measure and make sure your system is working correctly if you don't set up a suitable environment for consistent

progress. We'll discuss the best ways to stay consistent and the right way to track your body composition to ensure that you're making progress.

5. **The Application:** Knowledge is worthless if it's never applied or if you implement it incorrectly. Applying all the variables and science into a high-quality program that you can use in the real world is the whole reason for the previous parts of the system. Throughout this part of *Physique Secrets*, we'll cover how to apply everything we've discussed by designing a strength-training program and meal plan.

6. **The Progression:** Walking into the gym and kitchen with a program is the initial push to get moving in the right direction. You want to keep this momentum by staying consistent, progressing in strength and experience, and improving your body and programs. In this final part of *Physique Secrets*, we'll discuss the best methods for making progress and improvements in your training and nutrition and ensuring that your body is transforming through accurate tracking and measuring. This final part will help you avoid feeling like your results are taking you on a roller-coaster ride.

Every year, millions of fitness and nutrition books are sold, workout programs and nutrition plans are developed, supplements promising incredible results are manufactured, and millions of men actively try their hardest but fail to build their dream bodies.

In that same time frame and with the same available resources, thousands of average men from all walks of life and across a broad range of genetic capabilities are naturally building impressive physiques, proving that it is possible if done correctly.

The disconnect between getting and not getting results doesn't hinge on just one thing. You don't just do the wrong exercise or eat spinach instead of kale and have your results crumble.

It is a series of events that seem completely independent of each other yet add up to a bigger and bigger gap between the effort you put in and the results you get back.

It's like stacking dominoes. Each domino needs to be placed in line with the domino before it and the domino after it. A domino won't fall until the one before it falls, or if there's too large a gap between them.

This is the same problem I faced for the first six years of my journey, followed by three or four more years of understanding how to take overly scientific information and apply it to the real world.

This is also the exact reason why I wrote *Physique Secrets*—to help you avoid the years of failure and the years of studying and jump right into a proven order of events that everyone should follow to build the best physique possible as efficiently as possible and continue for life.

I have structured *Physique Secrets* to give you the exact order of events you need to follow. Each section and chapter of the book is in a specific order so that it builds on what came before, following a systematic approach.

All you need to do is use this system—which starts with flipping the page to the first part.

PART I

THE STRATEGY

SECRET 1

-

HOW TO CONSTRUCT AN AMAZING PHYSIQUE

CHAPTER 2

THE BLUEPRINT FOR AESTHETICS

Many men want a great body because it gives them more confidence, better health, more energy throughout the day, better sleep, more stability, fewer injuries and pain from daily tasks, better posture, less stress, and many other benefits.

The problem is that few people know how to get there. To make matters worse, many of those who think they know have an even deeper misunderstanding of what they need to do to build an impressive body.

Building an incredible body is similar to building anything else. It requires specific materials, a well-engineered framework for structural integrity, a sturdy foundation to build upon, a series of tasks completed in a particular order, and a lot of labor. Even though many different parts are required, everything comes together to form a cohesive structure.

When it comes to your body, the goal isn't just to create any old mediocre structure. You're reading this book because you want to create an amazing body, both inside and out.

This requires more than just eating your fruits and vegetables and going on a long walk. It takes a precise approach to create a genuinely aesthetic physique.

You can't build a great structure without a blueprint and detailed instructions to guide you.

Before you start, you must know where you are going and what you're trying to achieve. Without a clear end goal, you're going to waste a lot of time and energy working hard to make progress in the wrong direction.

So, to begin, let's outline a specific physique to work toward. This will provide a framework for the rest of the book and allow you to cut out anything that doesn't optimize your physique changes.

IT'S YOUR DREAM BODY

As someone who has worked with hundreds of men and women, I know that each person has a different dream body and end goal.

Your dream body is just that—it is yours and yours alone. After all, beauty is subjective.

You may not want a professional bodybuilder's physique that is extremely muscular and huge, but a lean body with just enough muscle for your shirts and pants to finally fit you properly.

So, when it comes to aesthetics, you will always have the final say on how you want to look based on your goals and preferences.

That is, as long as you have realistic expectations for what your body can achieve naturally.

Don't waste your time struggling to be Arnold Schwarzenegger or any of the steroid-enhanced bodybuilders you come across online when your natural genetic potential simply can't get you there.

You are training to be the best version of yourself. When you work toward having your dream body, you will be much happier with the results if you think about your own genetic potential and not the genetic lottery winners you see online.

However, this is all moot if it wreaks havoc on the rest of your body and your life in general.

Creating a fantastic physique on the outside is only one part of the equation. A genuinely incredible body functions just as well as it looks.

Building extensive amounts of muscle is worthless if you are constantly wiped out, injured, and unable to enjoy it. Reaching single-digit body fat levels is cool until you throw your health out the window or are always starving.

Instead, you should also look to optimize your health and how your body functions while improving your well-being, happiness, and confidence. Luckily, as you'll see, all of these improvements go hand in hand.

THE ONLY TWO THINGS THAT MATTER FOR CREATING AN AMAZING BODY

No matter what your dream body looks like, everything will come down to two key factors: fat loss and muscle building.

Through manipulating the amount of body fat that you have, along with the amount of muscle you build and the locations where you build this muscle, you'll be able to adjust the overall look and health of your body—and throughout this book, I will show you exactly how to do that.

Fat loss will be the primary determinant of how lean you are and will greatly improve many of your health markers. And building muscles is what allows you to accentuate specific areas of your body, look more chiseled and tight, appear more athletic, and adjust the shape and flow of your body.

However, in order to sculpt your body, you need an artist's chisel—i.e., the best methods of building muscle and losing fat.

Along with a high-quality diet, you need to do strength training. Strength training is the best method for consistently building muscle, vastly increasing your strength, rapidly leaning out, and improving your health and well-being, all at the same time.

We will discuss strength training in more detail later. Still, it's essential to understand that your nutrition program will be the primary determinant of your overall body size and weight, and your strength-training program will be the primary determinant of your overall body shape and the size of certain muscles (bone structure aside).

THE BENEFITS OF BEING LEAN AND MUSCULAR

Using strength training and a high-quality diet, my goal is to help you create the ultimate male body based on a combination of research and science, bodybuilding standards, professional athletes' functionality and aesthetics, and male preferences. With these things in mind, I have geared this book toward creating a specific physique—one that is lean, muscular, aesthetic, and incredibly strong.

It's the physique most men request and is often the most admired (and envied) body type. It's the body that looks like you know what you are doing when it comes to this whole fitness and nutrition thing.

Yet it's not just what your body looks like in swim trunks; it's the natural confidence and assurance that accompanies this body type.

It's the feeling and lifestyle of doing less work, enjoying your meals, having more time and energy to do the things you love to do, and still getting better results than the people training their butts off and sticking to a very strict diet.

I'm sure we've all known a guy this fit at one point or another. Whether you hated or admired him, we all wished we knew his secrets for success.

Throughout *Physique Secrets*, we will cover exactly what to do to improve every aspect of your body, both externally and internally. But, for right now, I want you to understand that building muscle and losing excess body fat can be highly beneficial for your health first, and for creating an amazing-looking body second.

Though this might be hard to stomach (pun intended), research has shown that being lean and having a decent amount of muscle is optimal for your health.[1] Being lean, as in not having a high level of body fat, protects you from developing diabetes, reduces the amount of chronic inflammation in your body, and improves your hormonal profile.[2] It also improves psychological well-being and reduces the risk of developing depression by up to 83 percent in some studies.[3]

It's no wonder that being lean is regarded as the number one method for increasing your longevity and staving off the effects of aging.[4,5,6]

Adding muscle mass to the equation compounds the health benefits. For example, increasing your muscle mass can lower your chronic inflammation levels, improve your sensitivity to insulin, reduce your risk of developing diabetes, improve your hormonal profile, and even increase your chances of surviving cancer.[7] Muscle mass also helps increase longevity and lessen the adverse effects of aging.[8]

So, being lean and muscular can benefit your health now and in the future.

To create an amazing physique, the first thing we will be looking to do is adjust your body fat percentage until your body can optimize your health markers, improve your hormone production, and process nutrients as well as possible.

The goal body fat percentage, based on many studies, is around 7%–12% body fat for optimal health. For reference, men in bodybuilding competitions have body fat percentages of 5%–6%, and men will typically start to develop extra belly fat at a body fat percentage of around 12%–15%.

So, getting to an optimal body fat percentage for your health will also help you create a lean physique that is tighter and denser, reveals your muscles, and helps you optimize your muscle building for faster and easier transformation.

THE MOST AESTHETIC PROPORTIONS AND MUSCLES

Knowing that building muscles and losing excess body fat can improve your body internally, you can concentrate on sculpting your body externally by reaching a specific aesthetic through targeted muscle growth.

Recent studies and surveys have shown that your proportions and symmetry matter most in defining an attractive physique. As long as your body meets certain ratios, your shoulder, waist, and chest sizes don't really matter.

The ratios that get the highest scores and are considered the most physically attractive include:[9]

- Waist circumference: about 45% of height

- Shoulder circumference: waist × 1.6

- Chest and back circumference: 10 to 12 inches (25 to 30 centimeters) greater than waist

- Upper-arm circumference: waist × 0.5

- Legs (including calf size): proportionate to upper body

As you can see from these recommendations, your shoulders will be wider than your chest, which will taper down to a skinny waist. Your arms will not be too small or too large but will complement your waist and upper-body thickness. And since the legs are often less important than the upper body for most males, your legs will simply need to match your upper body by being strong and muscular, though not overly huge or skinny.

This creates a proportionate body from top to bottom and a balanced physique from left to right, front to back, and muscle to muscle.

To achieve these proportions, you need to grow all of your major trainable muscles while dropping to a body fat percentage below 10%. This makes you look solid and aesthetic, yet still agile and athletic.

Your muscles will flow from one to the next with slight separation and possibly some striations. They will be dense and tight, not fluffy or disproportionate.

Specifically, the muscle groups will have these characteristics:

- **A wide upper back:** To achieve this, you want to target your latissimus dorsi (lats) and trapezius (traps). The lats should provide width and should form "wings" on your back that keep you from looking blocky. The lats will flow into a thick middle back formed by developing all three heads of the traps. The traps will tie in your neck, shoulders, lats, and lower back.

- **Broad shoulders:** This involves working all three heads of your deltoids—with extra attention to your lateral deltoids. The lateral deltoids will create "caps" on your shoulders, increasing your upper-body width and making your waist appear smaller.

- **Balanced, thick arms:** Target your biceps and triceps (the muscles in the front and back of your upper arm, respectively) to build strong, muscular upper arms that help fill out a T-shirt. Your triceps should be larger than your biceps, and your whole arm should be proportionate to every other muscle to avoid looking like Popeye.

- **A square chest:** You want your chest muscles to be square and broad while avoiding a "droopy" teardrop appearance. This involves developing your pectoral muscles, commonly known as the pecs. Keep the size of your chest muscles balanced with the size of your back and shoulders. If your chest muscles are overdeveloped, they will pull your shoulders forward.

- **Strong, muscular legs:** Achieving this requires targeting your gluteal muscles (glutes), hamstrings, quadriceps, and calves to achieve moderately sized legs that are proportionate to your upper body. Your legs should be strong and functional, yet big enough to extend your upper body's V taper into an X shape.

- **Well-defined abs:** Developing what we commonly refer to as a "six-pack" will involve targeting the exterior core muscles: the rectus abdominis and external oblique muscles.

- **A lean, tight waist:** Once you work on developing your upper body—your shoulders, upper back, and chest—a skinnier, tighter waist will come naturally, as long as you avoid overtraining your abs, which creates a blocky torso.

As you can see, everything is based on creating an aesthetic physique from head to toe and, most importantly, from the inside outward.

You're leaning out to improve your health markers, show off your muscles, and improve your muscle-building potential.

You're building muscle to improve your health markers and create a muscular and strong V taper with eye-catching proportions and symmetry.

You're strength training and eating the right things to accelerate your results while still being able to enjoy your life, become strong and balanced, improve your well-being, and not have to sacrifice your soul to the diet and gym devils.

Fortunately, you don't have to train for years and years to achieve all this. The major difference that more training experience brings to the table is greater overall muscle development and size.

This means that you can get an aesthetically pleasing body in as short a time as possible if you have a training program in which each training variable is optimized, an enjoyable nutrition program that helps you efficiently lose unwanted body fat while simultaneously building muscle, and the correct strength-training exercises to develop specific muscles.

CHAPTER 3

THE POWER OF
STRENGTH TRAINING

Building an impressive body doesn't happen overnight. And it definitely doesn't happen by coincidence.

Creating and growing muscles is a long-term process. Becoming impressively strong requires many months, but most likely years. How long it takes to get lean enough to see this muscle will depend on how much body fat you have now, but staying healthy and lean should be a lifelong goal.

Still, most men who lift weights or work out in the hope of looking phenomenal concentrate only on what they are doing in the moment or for that day. They are only concerned about that single workout session and how they can get the most out of it.

They are working out based on how they feel that day or what they look like day to day, versus week to week and month to month.

They might work hard and break a sweat through lifting weights, but there is no real structure and, in return, no real results.

The most common example—and I was guilty of doing it too—is for men to walk into the gym and make up a workout on the fly. They know they want to work a specific muscle group, so they just do a bunch of exercises that train that muscle group with many different intensities, set and rep schemes, and training techniques.

They fail to consider what exercises and weights they did last session or what they will do next session. Instead, it's all about the current workout. It's about how hard they worked today. How tired their muscles are today. How heavy they're breathing and how much they're sweating today.

This shortsighted approach is called exercising—doing a physical activity with little to no overarching structure, planning, or long-term progression.

If your goal is to work out, be healthy, and burn a few calories, then you can get away with simply exercising. However, this book isn't for you.

YOU'RE TRAINING, NOT EXERCISING

Physique Secrets' goal is to help you pack on muscle mass, become increasingly strong, and lean out using the most effective and efficient method. Accomplishing this takes a different approach and a specific method for working out: strength training.

Strength training is by far the best vehicle for getting you to your end goal and is what we will use to help you create an amazing body.

As you can probably understand, to truly be strength training, you need to be training to increase your strength. This requires two cohesive things: having a training program and working to improve your strength in one manner or another.

Training is performed with the purpose of satisfying a long-term goal. Therefore, it requires planning, time, and dedication to the goal you are training for.

Each training session is valuable because it places another domino in line to bring you one step closer to knocking down your final goal. Every improvement, no matter how minor, is an accomplishment.

By looking at the previous training session, you structure the current training session as part of a planned progression needed to continue to make improvements. You also consider the subsequent training sessions to ensure that progress is made and not lost because of a lack of foresight.

In the training process, workouts serve to improve performance measures like strength, endurance, or both. These workouts also cause metabolic and structural changes in the body, such as increases in muscle size.

Training is based on the fundamental biological concept that when physical stress is properly applied to your body, your body will adapt and improve. Our goal is to help our bodies make specific adaptations and physical improvements by applying stress in the form of strength training with weights, resistance, and machines.

To achieve the desired adaptations, you need to provide the correct stress followed by the perfect amount of recovery. Then you repeat the process at the peak of improvement before time is wasted or a return to pre-training status has begun.

However, you can't do this by just going to a gym, breaking a sweat, and chugging down a whey protein shake afterward.

Your body will adapt based on the exact stress it receives, and only in the areas stressed. Running 10 miles a day will stress your body and create adaptations, but they won't be the adaptations we are looking for.

This means you must gear your training toward specific goals and ensure that you stress specific muscles so you spur the exact improvements desired. This is referred to as training specificity.

In other words, to develop specific features and locations on your physique, you need to be specific in your training and diet programs to achieve the results you want. This takes a structured approach that you can only get from a training program.

As we've discussed, the changes and improvements we want from our training program are an increase in muscle size, also called muscular hypertrophy, followed by better strength, improved health, and fat loss.

You can achieve all these simultaneously by training to increase your strength. However, before diving deeper, let's understand what strength training entails.

DEFINING STRENGTH TRAINING

When it comes to fitness, you will find many terms that relate to strength training. You'll hear people use *resistance training*, *weight lifting*, *powerlifting*, *bodybuilding*, *power building*, and more to describe their workout methods or reasons for working out.

Strength training—which is a more specific form of resistance training—refers to using enough resistance, most often in the form of weights, to build strength by being able to handle more resistance, do more volume with the same resistance, or both.

Our goal is to build a specific body using our body weight, free weights (like dumbbells, barbells, kettlebells, etc.), or resistance from gym machines to increase our strength so that we increase our skeletal muscle size.

Strength training not only benefits your body physically by defining your most desired features to give you an aesthetic physique but also benefits your overall health and psychological well-being.

Here are just some of the health benefits of strength training:

- It improves your mental health and mood, reducing feelings of anxiety and depression.[1]

- It helps you cope with stress.

- It helps prevent chronic inflammation and heart disease.[2]

- It has been proven to improve quality of life by lowering causes of death like obesity.[3]

- Strength training improves your self-esteem, self-satisfaction, and self-concept, enabling you to stay socially active, which in turn relieves stress indirectly.[4]

- Studies also show that muscle mass can protect you against diabetes by helping to improve insulin sensitivity.[5,6]

There are many more that would make the above list extremely long. As you can see, a host of benefits come with strength training to develop an impressive physique. You can have all these benefits in addition to a well-sculpted body.

Plus, it's not too difficult to achieve. You don't need to spend a lifetime training to do so.

Still, it's important to realize that strength training is just a means to an end. The goal isn't to be good at strength training and lifting weights; it is to build an amazing body, both inside and out.

STRENGTH MEETS AESTHETICS

Strength training is the mechanism used to create an amazing body because it increases the size of your muscles. Though the muscles get larger and increase their cross-sectional area or total volume, they will be denser and appear much leaner and tighter.

This often leads to a debate in uneducated fitness circles about whether you should train for strength or for hypertrophy (muscle growth), as though the two were mutually exclusive.

These well-meaning folks don't understand that strength is a combination of morphological and neurological components. *Morphological* refers to the shape and size of the muscle. *Neurological* refers to the connection of the nerves to the muscles, which is better described as neuromuscular efficiency or neuromuscular coordination.

Strength and muscle building are two sides of the same coin. It's impossible to maximize one without the other.

There is an important saying about building muscles: if you're not getting stronger, you're probably not getting bigger.

More often than not, the stronger your muscles are, the more weight you can lift. The more weight you can lift, the more stress you can place on your muscles. The more stress you place on your muscles for extended periods, the larger your muscles will grow. The larger your muscles grow, the more weight they can generally lift—and the cycle starts again.

So, strength, muscle development, and building an exceptional body are all intertwined.

By training with the correct program variables and exercises, you can increase the exact muscles you want, in the exact locations you want, to create perfect proportions quickly.

Throughout *Physique Secrets*, we will discuss the proper way to train, progress, and improve strength. But even the best training program is worthless without a high-quality meal plan. They're like yin and yang—one without the other is just chaos.

CHAPTER 4

THE POWER OF
FLEXIBLE DIETING

You need both nutrition and strength training to build an amazing body. They work together to give you a strong, lean, muscular body.

Nutrition provides energy to fuel your training and the building blocks for muscle building. Strength training provides the correct stimulus for muscle development.

Your diet will also be the major determining factor behind your body-weight change. A quality diet with the correct nutrients and energy can make fat loss surprisingly easy.

However, the opposite is also true. It doesn't matter how hard you work or how good your strength-training program is if you don't know what to eat, how much to eat, and how to use what you know in the real world.

Nutrition is a huge topic that people spend years studying, and there always seems to be a new discovery or a random study that proves the best way to diet. You have people who swear by one diet, those who claim that diet didn't work for them, and yet another group of people who say no diet works for them.

The truth is that nutrition for losing fat quickly, gaining the perfect amount of muscle, and being healthy requires only a few guidelines based on what works in the real world, with real people, and is backed by high-quality, proven science.

A high-quality diet should be adjusted to work for you and not the other way around. It should be about including healthy and satiating foods instead of excluding foods that are deemed "unhealthy."

Your meal plan should prioritize weight change and building muscle through flexibility and proper nutrition programming.

THE REASON *DIET* IS A FOUR-LETTER WORD

The best meal plans and nutrition programs don't feel like diets. Instead, they become enjoyable routines that are easy to follow yet flexible when life happens.

Yes, the process can be easy and enjoyable when you know what you're doing and what is proven to work.

Why, then, do so many people struggle with the nutrition side of building their dream bodies? With two out of three people in the United States considered overweight and one in three considered obese, there is clearly a problem with the quantity and quality of foods being consumed.[1]

The skinny person who never seems to get hungry says, "You just need to become more mentally strong."

The supplement company says you don't need to change; you just need to buy their fat-burner and it will shed fat without any changes to your diet or exercise.

The overweight trainer tells you to eat a lot to fuel your training and to bulk up muscles, yet he never cuts back down to show off those muscles.

The roided-out bodybuilder who has dedicated his whole life to packing on muscle yet has never taken a nutrition course says to just eat chicken, broccoli, and rice and toughen up.

Eventually, after years of trying different strategies leading to your weight yo-yoing up and down, you will give up and think, *This whole diet thing isn't for me*—that you're just not meant to be lean and fit.

This is why *diet* has become a four-letter word that can send shivers down spines. Any mention of the word seems to immediately make people either hungry or anxious that breathing in too much air will break their progress.

How many times have you heard someone say, "I'm going on a diet," only to repeatedly break their diet as soon as it's snack time?

It's the lack of knowledge and know-how that makes getting lean and strong difficult and often even unhealthy when it should be increasingly healthy.

Dieting is as much a psychological process as it is physiological. Many research studies have shown that a lot of the problems associated with going on a diet are attributable to the placebo effect. The dieter believes he should be starving, feel miserable, and have little to no energy, so his body makes that happen.[2]

In reality, dieting doesn't affect mental energy or brain function—food restriction has actually been shown to possibly improve cognitive performance.[3] Skipping meals or eating very few calories doesn't cause blood sugar crashes and post-meal energy spikes—in fact, eating typically has the opposite effect and causes drowsiness.[4]

You don't need excess food to improve your mood, sleep well, have energy to complete tasks, or even train hard.[5]

The real reason for most failures is that people associate dieting with restriction. Cutting back and restricting yourself leads to a game of willpower versus hunger. Unless you are a robot with the willpower to say no forever, hunger and cravings always win. This is normal.

No self-help book on mental fortitude will be able to rid you of the constant fight between the food you want now and the body you want later. The battle between willpower and hunger will lead to unhappiness and eventual self-medication through eating comfort foods. Once this happens, getting back on your strict diet becomes much more challenging.

Sure, some people have more self-control than others and can stay on a strict diet or say no to their cravings for longer, but eventually, everyone breaks.

Plus, this isn't an enjoyable way to go through life. Shouldn't your dream body make you happy, not miserable?

Instead of having to rely on willpower, we will rely on a different approach to dieting. An approach that allows you to have your cake and eat it too.

Just imagine how much easier a diet will be if you can eat less but be just as full and satisfied while also building muscle and strength.

THE DIET TRIFECTA: STRUCTURE, BALANCE, AND FLEXIBILITY

Throughout the nutrition sections of *Physique Secrets*, we'll discuss how to create a flexible meal plan that gets results but doesn't feel like a "diet."

Flexible dieting helps you rid yourself of the black-or-white thinking associated with diet culture.

Foods aren't only healthy or unhealthy. There aren't strict times you need to eat. You don't have to choose between happiness and an amazing body. It's not a diet failure; it's a learning experience.

The goal of flexible dieting is to eat for weight change, muscle gain, and satiety (feeling sufficiently full). Everything else is a drop in the bucket or often leads to diet "failure."

The goal is to change from restriction and giving up foods to forming a healthy lifestyle that completely avoids the need for willpower. By switching from cutting out foods to adding foods that make you feel better, improve your body, and reduce your hunger, you will be more likely to stick with your nutrition program while enjoying the process.

You aren't avoiding any foods, like that ex-lover who you know is bad for you but is always available late at night when you're bored—you're increasing the foods that you know you will enjoy and that will put every other craving out of your mind.

Eating healthy, or at least certain foods, becomes part of your lifestyle, not a burden. You know that eating specific foods isn't mandatory but will fill you up and improve your life.

You can eat the other foods that you like, but you simply don't crave them as much when you know they aren't forbidden fruit.

If you make strength training and exercise part of your healthy lifestyle, you won't feel like a slave to your training program. Going to the gym won't be a time-consuming activity that takes forever to produce results.

Everything together will be enjoyable activity that helps you improve your health, energy levels, mental well-being, and more, with the added benefits of fat loss, and muscle and strength gains.

A high-quality nutrition program shouldn't feel like a diet. It should be flexible, balanced, and structured—not restrictive, monotonous, and uncontrolled.

It should be structured so you don't need to do calculations or guess at every meal. Instead, you have a routine that allows you to run on autopilot.

This structured approach doesn't cut out foods but is balanced with a variety of foods, offers multiple meal options, and is not overly restrictive.

Still, you can be flexible and make adjustments on the fly should life get in the way or your plans change. You can eat too much or too little here and there and not feel like a failure.

You're able to be flexible and jump right back into your diet afterward. It's the flexibility to make adjustments and allow yourself to "fail" without feeling like a failure and without stepping onto the slippery slope of repeated diet "failures."

This is how you will really succeed with dieting. You will be happier and healthier, with an amazing body to boot. Plus, it's not difficult to do.

Diet adherence does not need to be a constant struggle. Through structured, balanced, and flexible eating, you will see that you can still enjoy the food you eat, feel good, and see results.

In the upcoming sections, we will get into the science behind fat loss and how to apply different nutrition variables based on their order of importance. This will help you truly understand the minimal number of things you actually need to concentrate on to reel in the majority of the results you want.

By the end of *Physique Secrets*, you'll have the tools and knowledge necessary to stick to basic and proven eating methods while creating a diet that doesn't feel like a diet.

PART II

THE SCIENCE

SECRET 2

–

THE SIMPLE SCIENCE OF DEVELOPING MUSCLE AND STRENGTH

CHAPTER 5

THE FOUR PILLARS OF BUILDING MUSCLE

Most men know they can develop a strong and good-looking body by building specific muscles through strength training and eating well.

The problem and confusion arise when it comes to what to actually do to build muscles.

This confusion comes from a lack of understanding of the basics, which is caused by so-called experts in the fitness industry who give out half-baked information that both newcomers and experienced fitness trainees eat up.

Most people end up confused about whether they need to train with heavier loads or lighter ones, the numbers of reps and sets that are best, what they need to eat and in what quantities, how often they need to train to build muscle mass faster, whether to rest or not, when to rest, and for how long, etc., etc.

It's hard to get the body you want when you don't know what to believe and what to ignore. You have probably been pulled in so many directions that you don't even know up from down and left from right.

I understand this frustration, because I've been there too. I know the ups and downs and the endless cycle of information overload around building muscles.

Luckily, although the physiology of how muscles grow is complex, actually packing on muscle is not as complicated as this industry wants you to believe. Understanding the four fundamental pillars I'll talk about in this chapter is the key to building muscles effectively in almost every case.

These pillars will provide the structure for your strength-training and nutrition programs. Each pillar is needed to hold up the rest of the book and deliver results. If even one of these pillars is ignored, the others won't be able to stand, and your structure will collapse.

But if you apply these four pillars, your muscles will grow bigger, stronger, and faster than you can imagine.

PILLAR #1: PROVIDING THE CORRECT STIMULUS (STRENGTH TRAINING)

If you want to build muscle and strength, you first need to give your muscles and body a reason to want or need to grow—a spark to start the fire, so to speak.

To accomplish this, you must put the muscles you want to grow under a new stress that is specific to the improvements you want to see. Then you need to repeat this process with enough volume, intensity, and frequency to ensure maximal growth without compromising your results.

But within this process, there are different combinations of sets, reps, training loads, repetition speeds, and rest periods that will dictate the progress you make.

In other words, it's not about providing a stressor or stimulus; it's about providing the correct stimulus for efficient results.

To optimize muscle-building results, it is crucial to consider three main factors:

1. Mechanical tension

2. Muscle damage

3. Metabolic stress

When you are strength training, your muscles will experience mechanical tension, which can lead to muscle damage and create metabolic stress depending on how you train.

This has led a generation of old-school bodybuilders to assume that since a muscle pump feels and looks awesome, they get sore the next day, they are training very hard, and they know that stress on their muscles leads to larger muscles, then all three of these mechanisms must create muscle growth.

This logic shaped their workouts to train one muscle group a day, train each muscle group once a week, do a lot of sets for that single muscle group, take shorter rest periods, and do around 12 reps per set.

Unfortunately, just because your muscles swell up and look awesome in the middle of a workout or get sore the next day doesn't mean it's causing muscle growth.

That's why you will follow what research has proven and work toward maximizing mechanical tension and minimizing both muscle damage and metabolic stress.

Let's take a closer look and discuss what each means for training in the real world.

Rule #1: Prioritize Mechanical Tension

To create mechanical movement, a nerve impulse (electrical signal) from your brain is sent to your spinal cord and then to your muscles. This causes a cascade of metabolic processes within your muscle fibers.

The contractile units inside your muscle fibers create tension, then contract and shorten the muscle. This pulls on your tendons and rotates your bones around your joints, causing mechanical movements.

When the mechanical tension is high, such as when you're lifting weights or strength training, the structural integrity of your muscle fibers is compromised. To create more force and handle more tension in the future, your body will improve the exact fibers that were stressed, and will do so in a way specific to the stress that was applied.

Our goal is to increase the size of the muscle fibers in specific muscles, i.e., cause muscle growth.

High and prolonged mechanical tension is the primary stimulus for muscle growth. It is the one thing that has been proven to tell your body to grow your muscles.[1]

Now, as you might have noticed, the primary trigger for your body to grow your muscles isn't just mechanical tension; neither is it heavy or high mechanical tension. Instead, it is a high and prolonged mechanical tension.

When it comes to training, high mechanical tension is most often the amount of weight you are lifting, while prolonged tension is the time spent under tension—or the total number of reps performed with a weight.

So, in other words, to create the most mechanical tension on your muscles and, in turn, grow your muscles in the most efficient way possible, you will want to lift weights that are as heavy as possible for as long as possible. Rinse and repeat.

This is very important to know and understand because it will provide the foundation for all your training variables.

To put the most tension on your whole muscle, you need to make sure you work it through its full range of motion and create tension both when the muscle is flexed and when it is stretched. This will trigger two different growth mechanisms: active and passive tension.

Active tension is created when your muscles are actively working to contract and shorten, the way a bicep does when you curl your arm upward.

Passive tension occurs when your muscles are slowly releasing tension, like when you lower your arm back down from a biceps curl. The tension is caused by friction between the contractile units in your muscles.

You can picture it like trying to hold a rope during a tug-of-war but not being able to get a strong enough grip and ending up with rope burn on your palms from the friction.

Studies indicate that exercises that involve both active and passive movements are superior to those that involve purely active or passive training alone when it comes to maximizing strength and muscle mass.[2,3,4]

The goal is to provide sufficient mechanical tension by finding the right balance between lifting very heavy weights and doing enough repetitions to give the muscles enough time under tension and volume to grow.

We will get into exactly how to do this when we discuss each optimal strength-training variable in an upcoming section.

Rule #2: Minimize Muscle Damage

When the structural integrity of your muscle fibers is compromised, the fibers can become microscopically damaged, and microtears can occur inside them. This possible muscle damage is not large enough to cause injury, but it is stressful enough to trigger a response from your body.

If you've been to the gym before or performed any exercise, even with just your body weight, you've probably experienced some degree of soreness. It's not unusual to hobble out of bed or struggle to hoist yourself off the couch the day after a workout.

Although getting sore after strength training is normal, you need to understand that soreness and damaged muscles do not equate to results. Excessive muscle damage can prevent you from training as hard or as often as you otherwise would, which in turn hinders muscle growth.[5] As a result, muscle growth is impaired because you compromise mechanical tension, which is the primary stimulus for muscle growth. And damaged muscles need more time to heal and repair before they can grow, which also slows muscle growth.

Therefore, as you train, getting as sore as possible and breaking down your muscles as much as possible shouldn't be your goal.

Instead of focusing on performing tons of exercises and reps, focus on what you can do to achieve more mechanical tension while minimizing muscle damage. This might even include doing less work during one training session so you can increase tension in those same muscles in future workouts.

Rule #3: Minimize Metabolic Stress

If you have ever trained very hard before, you most likely experienced a burning sensation in your muscles. That burning feeling is the result of what's called "metabolic stress."

When your muscles need rapid bursts of energy that can't be replenished fast enough through the use of oxygen, such as during strength training, hydrogen ions (H+) accumulate and create an acidic environment inside your cells.

As your muscles keep creating energy, more hydrogen ions and other metabolites accumulate in your muscle cells faster than your muscles can clear them. This leads to metabolic stress, a burning feeling, and reduced muscle function.

Metabolic stress is simply the result of your body not being able to generate enough energy, pump oxygen into your muscles, and clear negative waste products of chemical reactions in your muscles. Basically, it's stress in your muscles caused by metabolic reactions and processes.

It's like if a bunch of orders for the newest Apple iPhone come in too quickly and the orders can't be filled fast enough, so they start to get backed up, the website crashes, and Apple doesn't have enough truck drivers to deliver the product.

This is also why you get a "pump" in your muscles. Because your muscles are under constant tension when you work out a specific muscle with incomplete recovery, blood and oxygen can't be cleared out of your muscles after a set, making them appear larger and "pumped up."

Although many people love the pump, metabolic stress can affect your training intensity and muscle growth. It increases fatigue, causing you to perform fewer repetitions and lift less weight, which may hinder mechanical tension.[6]

If you have ever trained before, I'm sure it's easy to understand how that burning feeling can stop you from being able to maximize mechanical tension.

And just so you don't come for my throat, metabolic stress happens naturally, but it hasn't been proven to lead to muscle growth. It was just thought to help because it occurred naturally when there was mechanical tension. It was kind of like arguing about whether the chicken or the egg came first. Just like with muscle damage, we will also want to reduce metabolic stress for optimal muscle growth.

So, when training for muscle growth, you will have to consider these three factors: increasing mechanical tension while minimizing muscle damage and metabolic stress.

In an upcoming section, we'll discuss how each of the variables that go into creating an optimized strength-training program will follow these three factors.

PILLAR #2: PROGRESSIVELY AND CONSISTENTLY OVERLOAD YOUR MUSCLES

As you strength train, your muscle strength increases, and you adapt to the current stress. Your muscles need a slightly larger amount of stress to trigger further adaptations.

This is what is referred to as progressive overload. This principle states that you need to progressively increase your muscles' working load to continually challenge your body and muscles with new stimuli to adapt and respond to. If your muscles aren't progressively overloaded, they will stop improving.

When it comes to creating mechanical tension in your muscles so they can keep growing from workout to workout and month to month, you need to keep increasing the mechanical tension inside your muscle fibers by manipulating certain training variables.

In general, there are two main ways in which you can increase mechanical tension:

1. You can increase the amount of weight you're using while keeping the total time/ distance you're lifting the weight the same.

2. You can increase the amount of time/distance you're lifting the weight while keeping the amount of weight you're using the same.

In other words, to build muscles, you will need to build strength by either increasing the resistance that you're using or increasing the muscles' time under tension.

Increasing the load or resistance your muscles have to work against is the best way to progressively overload them. Most often, this is done by lifting heavier weights. This allows you to progress nicely and build more muscle for a better-looking and -operating body.

The second way to consistently increase the amount of mechanical tension your muscles feel is to lengthen the amount of time they are under resistance. This is done by increasing the total number of repetitions in the workout. By performing more reps, you increase the amount of time your muscles are under tension while also using active and passive tension.

Research has found that lifting lighter weights for a longer time leads to the same muscle growth as lifting heavier weights for a shorter time, as long as the same total volume is present.[7]

One method emphasizes more repetitions or time under tension, and the other emphasizes weight.

Consistently and progressively increasing the weight you lift and/or the reps you perform will lead to consistent muscle growth.

That being said, it's safer for a beginner to focus more on increasing the time under tension than on using heavier weights. Therefore, start by lifting lighter weights but performing more reps. You can then move on to lifting heavier weights when your muscles are strong enough that you can lift heavy weights comfortably without letting your form deteriorate.

PILLAR #3: PROVIDE THE RIGHT BUILDING BLOCKS (NUTRITION)

Building muscles is like building a house. If you have the desire to build the house, the need for it, enough money, and a location, then you will start building.

When you're building your house, you need to have all the materials in the correct quantities and enough people and energy to complete the job. If you don't buy any wood or you run out of wood, you won't be able to build your house. Likewise, your house won't go up if you don't have enough manpower to put up the walls, install the plumbing, wire the electrical, and complete the task.

This is analogous to giving your muscles the right kind and amount of nutrients to grow. So, what does your body actually need to build muscle?

The truth is, muscle is just a dumb piece of meat. It doesn't take a genius or a degree in nutrition to build muscles. It's all about having the correct stimulus and nutrients.

In 1982, a group of researchers wanted to find out what makes up human muscle tissue. To do this, they had the awful (or awesome, depending on your perspective) job of cutting up some cadavers.[8]

They were able to determine that all human muscle tissue is composed of three things:

- Protein

- Energy, specifically glycogen and triglycerides

- Lots of water

As you can see, these three things your body uses and needs for muscle growth are relatively easy to consume in a diet. Let's take a brief look at each of them.

Building Block #1: Proteins

Proteins are made up of smaller units known as amino acids, which your body rearranges and combines to create new proteins and other molecules.

There are a total of 20 amino acids in proteins. Your body can make all but 9 of these amino acids by rearranging the atoms of other amino acids already in your body.

Therefore, it is essential that you consume these 9 amino acids in your diet, which is why they are called essential amino acids (EAAs).

A good portion (over 40%) of the body's protein is found in structural components such as muscles, bones, teeth, skin, tendons, hair, nails, and more. These proteins provide structure, support, and movement for your body.

Over 25% of the protein in your body is found in your organs, while the rest is spread throughout your blood.

These proteins create antibodies that help your body fight infections; hormones that act as chemical messengers; buffers to help regulate your body's pH (acid-base balance); enzymes that influence the rate of chemical reactions that take place in your cells; and transporters that bind and carry substances like vitamins and minerals in and out of your body's cells.

Proteins, specifically amino acids, are the building blocks of muscle. If you don't consume enough of all the building blocks, you will not build muscle.

This means that you have to eat all 9 essential amino acids, and you need enough of each of them to give your muscles the building blocks they require. Also, the other 11 amino acids, though nonessential and able to be created in our bodies, are important to consume, since the various amino acids work synergistically to improve processes in our bodies.

When it comes to eating protein, this is something that you can base an eating plan around with little difficulty—no need to overcomplicate it.

So, it doesn't matter if you're trying to get to single-digit body fat levels or pack on 20 pounds of mass—you will be able to eat enough protein to build muscle with little worry.

Building Block #2: Energy (Glycogen and Triglycerides)

Building muscles is a very energy-intensive process. Luckily, your body not only obtains energy directly from the food you eat but stores energy as well, so it has a lot of energy ready to use.

Energy in the form of glucose gets stored as glycogen, and fatty acids as triglycerides.

Glycogen is made up of highly branched chains of glucose, and it is stored in the liver and skeletal muscles. Due to its structure, glycogen can be broken down quickly into glucose to give your body energy when it needs it.

Triglycerides and fatty acids make up 95% of the fat that you eat and are stored around your body as body fat.

As long as you are nowhere near essential body fat levels, which are around 3% in men,[9] and your body doesn't need to break down its own tissue to survive, you will have enough stored glucose and fatty acids to metabolize in order to fuel the process of building muscle and moving.

In fact, a man with around 6% body fat and weighing 190 pounds (86 kilograms) will have over 48,000 stored calories that can be broken down for processes in his body. Though many people consider this as "having almost no fat," there is still plenty of energy to build pounds of muscle.

This isn't even considering that you will still be eating and drinking energy. Later we'll go over how to keep supplying your body with the proper number of calories for muscle building and fat loss.

As we will discuss, eating enough calories during the day will help you build more muscle and, in turn, will have a very beneficial effect on fat loss as well. This means you can simplify your diet plan in order to consume just enough energy or calories.

Building Block #3: Water

Water and hydration are topics that many people want to complicate, but I am going to make them very simple.

Water constitutes a greater percentage of your body mass than any other substance. It helps fill the spaces inside and outside the cells and in all major vessels.

This is why water is often considered the most important nutrient. It is the only nutrient we can't survive without for even a few days. In fact, dehydration caused by water loss amounting to more than 7% of your body weight can lead to death.[10]

When it comes to building muscles, no matter your diet, you can drink as much water as you need. It's very easy to add a glass or two of water to a meal plan to supply your body and muscles with enough water for metabolic processes.

The bottom line is that as long as you have the stimulus to tell your body to build muscle (i.e., a strength-training program) and consume these three building blocks, you can and will have the necessary ingredients to support the muscle-building process. You don't need to make it more complicated than that.

Now that we've covered the first three pillars of muscle building, let's look at how your body converts stimuli and building blocks into beautiful muscle.

PILLAR #4: MAXIMIZE RECOVERY

If you are a fitness or bodybuilding enthusiast, odds are you've heard the old bodybuilding saying "Muscles aren't built in the gym."

Though this is accurate from a bird's-eye view, it's not as easy as chugging down a protein shake post-workout and letting your body get to work growing your muscles.

Many gym-goers spend an unnecessary amount of time trying to hack their training and diet programs. They look up videos, read clickbait articles, train excessively hard, and are very strict with their diets, almost to the point of obsessiveness.

Yet few people ever reap the benefits of all this hard work. They often don't give their muscles enough time to recover and don't give them the best environment for recovery.

It's like wasting all your money on the car of your dreams but never being able to drive it. The car is there, you did all the work to afford it, you just can't ever use it. What was the point of all the hard work if you missed the last detail that makes owning your dream car enjoyable?

Most people overlook the concept of recovery because they have the wrong impression of how training helps the body build muscle and strength. Yet recovery plays a vital role in the muscle-building process.

In addition, recovery is often a very passive thing. Training and dieting take lots of noticeable effort, and both are tangible. You can feel and be aware of the exact amount of each that you are doing.

Recovery, on the other hand, is difficult to feel and frequently becomes a back-of-mind thing that takes a backseat to training and nutrition once a person leaves the gym.

It seems weird to many active individuals that doing less can be better for building muscle and losing fat. But being "lazy" might help you look better, feel better, and be healthier.

Regular strength training is key to peak physical fitness and muscle growth. But if you want to get the most out of your training, you will need to provide your body with the proper environment to recover from your training and synthesize muscle proteins.

This means knowing and doing what science has shown gives your muscles and body the best environment to recover. These factors include:

- Time

- Sleep

- Stress reduction

- Proper nutrition

In the following sections, we'll talk about how to get the most out of each of these, but for now, let's just talk briefly about each one so you can set up the last pillar of your muscle-building plan. We will start with arguably the most important part of your recovery process: time.

Recovery Rule #1: Provide Adequate Time

As you know now, strength training causes metabolic stress and damage to your muscle fibers. This leads to an inflammatory response, sometimes soreness, and a complex process of repairing any damage created and building new muscles while changing the internal structure to function better in the future.

How long it takes your body to fully recover, including growing new muscles, depends on how much damage and stress you put it through during training. If you put a muscle group through a very intense training session, with very heavy weights and a substantial number of sets, that muscle group will require a much longer recovery time than a muscle group that did only a few sets.

To a certain extent, you want to provide the perfect amount of stimulus for growth and the perfect amount of time for growth and recovery. Too much recovery time and you're limiting your growth potential. Too little recovery time and you're digging too large a recovery hole to climb out of, which often leads to overtraining or just poor results.

Overtraining causes decreased strength, plateaued muscle growth, and injuries. And if you continue training too hard without proper recovery, you can experience complete hormonal dysfunction and a downturn in overall well-being.

On the other hand, letting your muscles continue to rest when they are fully recovered means they're missing the opportunity to begin the growth process again. This leaves you with less muscle growth than you could have.

Instead, you need to allow just enough recovery time so you neither overtrain nor undertrain. Adequate recovery time takes many factors into account.

Throughout this book, we'll talk about the best ways to train to build muscle and lose fat. We will also discuss how to create the perfect nutrition program to maximize your results.

All your training variables come together to create a perfect program and determine how much recovery time your muscles will need between training sessions. Your training experience and genetics will also play a role in how quickly you fully recover.

Finally, the amount of sleep you get in a night, your chronic stress levels, and the quality of your diet will also affect how intensely you can train and how long your recovery period will take. Let's discuss these three factors next, starting with sleep.

Recovery Rule #2: Get Enough Sleep

Sleep serves many vital functions in the human body, including muscle recovery and growth. Getting enough high-quality sleep can have substantial effects on your muscle-building and fat-loss outcomes.

Studies show that sleep deprivation steps up the activity of degradation pathways and lowers the activity of protein synthesis pathways.[11] In other words, the systems in your body that break down nutrients and structures become more active, and the systems that build protein structures are less active than usual. This directly inhibits muscle growth and can even cause muscle loss.

But if you get enough sleep, your body releases enough growth and anabolic hormones for tissue growth and muscle repair, which in turn aids muscle recovery and growth. It also revs up protein synthesis pathways, creating significant stimuli for muscle growth.

To simplify, a long-term research study showed that improving your sleep can lead to pounds of muscle gained and pounds of fat lost over a year, even without exercise or dieting.[12]

So, if you are looking to increase muscle mass, drop body fat, and change your body composition, you need to get enough high-quality sleep, which we'll discuss how to do later in the book.

Recovery Rule #3: Reduce Stress Levels

Almost all research studies have shown that stress generally has negative effects on your body, including a greater likelihood of dying sooner.[13] Stress can affect many parts of your life, like your ability to build muscle, process food, get stronger, keep food cravings at bay, lose fat, and recover after a workout.

One study found that having a lot of psychological stress doubled the length of time it took participants to recover compared to having low psychological stress. The high-stress group's recovery was impacted for over 96 hours after a moderate strength-training workout.[14]

If you can recover from your training at only half the speed or half the capacity you should be able to, you will have a hard time creating an amazing body. This isn't even getting into the effects stress has on body fat storage and the processing of nutrients.

So, as you can see, stress from work, life, family, and other struggles can take a toll on your training and drag you backward—by several miles—in your journey toward achieving your desired physique.

Therefore, if you are super-stressed, doing hard, high-intensity training may not be the best way to relieve the stress. Instead, it's likely to create a recovery hole you would need an excavator to dig yourself out of.

To avoid the detrimental effects that stress may have on your training and goals, you will want to do all it takes to prevent or at least manage stress, which we'll talk about later in the book.

Recovery Rule #4: Follow a Proper Diet

At this point, you already know that muscles need to be fed a proper diet in order to grow. Specifically, you need to consume enough protein, water, and energy.

In general, if you eat a healthy diet and take in the three building blocks of muscle, you will give your body the best chance to recover and build muscle after a workout. This includes muscle, bone, tendon, ligament, and neural (nervous system) recovery, as your diet (and everything else discussed in this pillar) can improve recovery capacity and reduce the time needed for recovery.

However, when it comes to musculoskeletal and neuromuscular recovery, research has identified what you should factor into your diet.[15] In an upcoming section, I'll help you place these into a meal program:

- Enough protein (duh)

- Omega-3 fatty acids

- Anti-inflammatory foods such as fruits and vegetables

- Gut-health-improving foods that are high in fiber, and possibly foods that contain probiotics

As you can see, it comes down to eating healthy foods and sticking to a few nutritional staples. By eating healthy and getting enough of the foods our bodies need to build muscle, your body will be able to process nutrients optimally to speed up recovery. We'll discuss nutrient processing in the "pillars of weight change."

◇◇◇

Building muscle is a highly complex process involving many different functions and changes in the body. If I tried to describe all these, this book would have another several hundred pages.

The good news is that you don't need to be scientifically brilliant to have a functional understanding of research findings on muscle growth or to be able to use the information to gain muscle.

These four fundamental pillars form the foundation of this understanding. Just stimulate your muscles by overloading them with heavy enough tension for a long enough period of time while avoiding excessive damage and metabolic stress during the workout.

Then feed your muscles and allow them time to repair and build new and more muscles after the workout, and you will be able to completely transform your body. In upcoming sections, we'll break down exactly how to do this in the best way possible.

CHAPTER 6

THE MOST COMMON MUSCLE-BUILDING MISTAKES MEN KEEP MAKING

In this chapter, I'll tackle some of the beliefs and mistakes that prevent a lot of men from getting the most out of their training and diet—specifically when it comes to gaining muscle and strength.

Unfortunately, many fitness coaches have made millions of dollars by spreading these myths or even outright lies. This leads to many men repeatedly making the same mistakes when it comes to their training and diet.

If you have read the previous chapters and understand most of the information, you will notice that most of the myths that I present, and that you have more than likely believed, are easily debunked using the pillars of building muscle.

The important thing to understand is that most of the false information starts with a simple proven concept that is manipulated in an effort to either outsmart science or create a new and fancy concept, program, or product to sell. Instead of following what is proven, people are led astray by myths and lies that slow their muscle-building progress or even bring it to a grinding halt.

This chapter could be hundreds of pages long, but let's go over the biggest and most common mistakes men make that could prevent you from maximizing your muscle and strength gains.

BELIEVING YOU CAN'T BUILD MUSCLE AND LOSE FAT SIMULTANEOUSLY

People are often misled by the belief that you have to choose between being lean or building muscle, which completely changes how you will eat and train.

The thinking is that if you're losing fat because you are eating fewer calories than you're burning in a day, your body won't build muscle because it will need to conserve energy. So, if you want to gain muscle, you have to be willing to say goodbye to your abs and "bulk up" to finally have enough calories to build muscle.

But it is definitely possible to gain muscle and lose body fat simultaneously, because your body can direct nutrients to muscle mass and fat mass independently.

Just imagine how much worse off humans would be if our bodies couldn't perform protein synthesis unless we were in a calorie surplus. Every time we got injured, our bodies would just wait until we ate enough before starting to heal.

Many studies and real-world people's experiences conclusively prove that muscle gain and fat loss can happen concurrently. For example, a study was conducted on overweight people who started a strength-training program. After training for 12 weeks, the participants had gained about 9 pounds of muscle mass and lost close to 9.5 pounds of body fat.[1] That's only a half-pound weight change but a completely different body composition.

Hundreds of studies on lean and overweight, young and old, healthy and unhealthy, and male and female participants have conclusively shown that you can build muscle and lose fat simultaneously.[2,3]

With an optimized strength-training program and correct nutrition, even elite athletes and professional bodybuilders can build muscle and lose fat at the same time.[4] In fact, losing fat while gaining muscle, known as body recomposition, should almost always be the goal of any high-quality program.

TRAINING AND EATING DIFFERENTLY BECAUSE OF YOUR BODY SHAPE (SOMATOTYPE)

Since a highly discredited research study was conducted in the 1940s, the fitness and nutrition industries have clung to the myth that you need to eat or train differently based on your body shape. This is called somatotyping.

In somatotyping, there are three main types of body shapes: ectomorphic (skinny and tall), endomorphic (bulky), and mesomorphic (athletic and fit).

Thinking that you fit into a specific body type makes sense and has been shown to be a good predictor of athletic performance, and there are plenty of "bro science" training programs that hang their hats on this idea.

But the truth of the matter is that somatotypes give your body a description at a particular point in time. Your current body shape has nothing to do with the physiology of your muscles and can never predict how your muscles will respond to your training.

In one study, researchers found that people of the same body type had completely different muscle gain and fat loss after training for 12 weeks compared with other people with the same body type.[5] Furthermore, there was no correlation between their muscle gain, fat loss, and starting somatotype.

In reality, your somatotype is just a watered-down version of your current body-fat-to-muscle-mass ratio.

Mesomorphy basically means having a large amount of muscle mass. Endomorphy comes down to body fat percentage and being weak compared to your weight. Ectomorphy is the opposite of endomorphy but relates more to height, so you are weak compared to your height.

In fact, the reason you might fall into a specific somatotype is because of your diet, not your genetics. For example, you might be an endomorph due to a poor diet and a higher body fat percentage, not because you were born an endomorph.

The only thing somatotyping does is tell you how many calories you need to eat to lose fat or gain muscle. There is no magical percentage of macronutrients that changes based on your body shape and somatotype.

BELIEVING YOU DON'T HAVE THE GENETICS TO GAIN A LOT OF MUSCLE

A famous study was done in which participants were told that they were being given steroids to test the steroids' effects. During the study, the strength of the participants in the steroid group skyrocketed by two- to threefold compared with that of the "normal" group.[6] The steroid group developed more muscle mass and even lowered their body fat percentage by the end of the study. This is pretty normal for people on steroids when compared with people who are natural.

That is, if you're actually given steroids. But no participants in this study were given steroids; they were only told they were given steroids.

The study wasn't to test the effects of steroids but to test the effects of psychologically believing you can achieve something.

Many studies have shown that when people are told that they genetically can't do something, no matter how hard they try, their subconscious efforts result in a self-fulfilling prophecy.

The truth is that we all have limits to how much muscle we can gain based on our body structure and other physiological variables, but this doesn't mean you can't gain muscle at all.[7]

Also, where you currently are in terms of your physique and the amount of muscle mass you have does not predict the amount of muscle you can develop. Studies have shown that your baseline muscle mass is not a good predictor of the results you can or will achieve.[8]

Your genetics are influential, but they don't stop you from gaining enough muscle to change your physique's overall appearance and aesthetic.

While you might have a different end result and need to adjust your expectations, it's important to understand that research has conclusively proven that every man can develop a truly incredible physique if he has the correct diet and training program.

In other words, your current body isn't a life sentence, and it doesn't predict how your body will look after you start a quality training program.

AVOIDING HEAVY WEIGHT LIFTING

When it comes to training, weight lifting is one of the most beneficial methods for creating positive changes in your body. It is easily accessible for most populations and lets you follow the most research-backed strategies for training to build muscles.

All in all, research has proven that the best way to make your body internally the best that it can be is through heavy resistance training, and the most conducive method of providing heavy resistance, for most populations, is through weight lifting.[9]

Weight lifting is one of the few ways to train that allows you to consistently overload your body with more and more weight. It also lets you follow your proper body mechanics and gives you many options for changing exercises to fit your body and work different muscles from different angles.

Weight lifting even results in fewer injuries than almost every other athletic activity, including CrossFit, team sports, running, powerlifting, and more.[10]

It's kind of a "jack-of-all-trades" and master of building muscles. That's why professional athletes, the world's strongest people, senior citizens, and fitness models all train using weights.

The best benefits come from lifting heavy weights. Heavy weight lifting and strength training helps:

- Your bones, tendons, and ligaments get stronger and denser, which helps prevent injuries.

- Your muscles coordinate better, improving your balance and overall coordination.

- Your body burn more calories throughout the day and increase your fat loss.

- Release beneficial hormones for muscle growth, fat loss, less anxiety, and happier moods.

- Build strength and muscle mass much faster.

- Enhance fat loss, burn more calories, become leaner, and have more developed muscles.

- Suppress hunger so you can lose unwanted fat far more easily and avoid overeating after training.

Doing cardio, using equipment like resistance bands, or doing body-weight exercises is excellent. Still, these will never give you the same consistent results as using free weights, cables, or well-designed machines.

PRIORITIZING EXPENSIVE GYM MACHINES, BANDS, OR OTHER FANCY EQUIPMENT

To build beautiful muscles, you don't need thousands of dollars, fancy gym equipment, machines, or any expensive contraption.

Each year, some new and fancy gym equipment or expensive workout class is "specifically designed" to beat the time-honored methods that have been used for decades. You're made to believe that the equipment you use or the gym you go to is way more important than the basics of strength training.

In reality, you will get better results by sticking to the tried-and-true free weights—like the dumbbell, barbell, pull-up bar, and possibly cable machines. Many studies have demonstrated that free weights can give you better results—even up to 30% more muscle gains[11,12]—than most gym machines. Free weights provide excellent tissue stress distribution, resulting in the activation of more muscles, which in turn results in more strength development and muscle growth.[13] They follow a strength curve that is closer to your normal biomechanics, you don't lose tension in your muscles like you often do with bands and fancy exercises, it is easier to progress properly and follow a program, you aren't locked into an exact movement pattern, and you can do a full range of motion on most exercises to stress your muscles completely.

Your muscles are built to work in the real world and perform specific movements. Trying to add fanciness often just works against your normal biomechanics and becomes a waste of your time, money, and energy.

TRAINING EXCESSIVELY HARD IN THE NAME OF BUILDING MORE MUSCLE FASTER

The idea that "more is better" and "no pain, no gain" ends up holding more people back than getting them better results faster.

How hard you train and how sore your muscles get don't directly correlate to the amount of muscle you will build. In fact, excessive muscle soreness could be a sign of overtraining, not getting enough nutrients, or even a serious injury, but not that more muscle is being built.

When you train to completely annihilate your muscles by causing extensive muscle damage, metabolic stress, and fatigue, you shoot yourself in the foot for the rest of the workout and even for future workouts.

Muscle damage and metabolic stress prevent you from lifting as much weight. This is because there are fewer contractile units in your muscles that can help you lift, and metabolic waste products stop your muscles from contracting. And the longer you work out, the more fatigued your muscles and nerves become, making them less coordinated and less effective. This leads to less weight lifted and makes it much more likely that you'll hurt yourself by using bad technique.

Once that training session ends, you have dug such a deep recovery hole that your muscles might not be able to recover fully by the next session.

Once you have stimulated a muscle to grow, adding more sets and reps will have little effect on muscle growth, but it will significantly affect fatigue and recovery.

In other words, you need to stimulate your muscles, not annihilate them.

It's like filling a bucket with water. Once the bucket is full, adding more water will overflow the bucket and cause other problems for you.

Don't let your ego and drive to outwork science overrule a high-quality program that keeps you progressing consistently and effectively.

DOING AS MANY DIFFERENT EXERCISES AS POSSIBLE TO HIT EVERY MUSCLE FIBER IN A SINGLE MUSCLE

There is a common belief that to develop a muscle to its full potential, you need to do a ton of variations of the same exercise to hit every fiber in the muscle.

It is true that there are a ton of different angles and different lengths of muscle fibers in a single muscle.[14] Muscle fibers are also separated into units of nerves, known as motor units, that allow the muscle to contract different fibers separately.

With different lengths, angles, and motor units, you can activate different regions or locations of a muscle at a time. You can also train different areas of a single muscle more intensely than other areas by using specific exercises.[15,16]

Muscle activation often leads to muscle growth, so it is possible to use certain exercises to target specific locations in a muscle for growth.

However, doing a lot of slight variations will mostly hinder your muscle growth instead of building more muscle.

First, it will lead to excessive fatigue, resulting in worse muscle growth as you continue to add exercises.

Next, many fibers in a single muscle are very similar and help perform the same movements and functions. So, if you lift a heavy enough weight and come close enough to technical failure (when your technique starts to suffer), your body will need to call upon as many muscle fibers as are available to perform that movement or exercise. It doesn't matter if the fibers aren't perfectly aligned with that movement or are better stressed by another movement.

Doing slightly different exercises will give you a different feel neurologically, but the same muscle fibers will often be trained and possibly overtrained.

So, you will probably get better results if you use a single exercise for each specific muscle function and ensure that there is enough tension to work all the muscle fibers. Then you should progress with that exercise before adding more exercises or switching to a different one.

FREQUENTLY CHANGING UP YOUR PROGRAM AND EXERCISES BEFORE YOU'VE MAXIMIZED YOUR STRENGTH AND MUSCLE GAINS

How many times have you heard that doing the same exercise multiple times is bad for your gains because your muscles become accustomed to it and stop growing? Instead, the theory goes, you need to "shock" and "confuse" your muscles with new exercises and programming so they keep growing.

Except muscles are just dumb pieces of meat. They can't be "confused" or "shocked" by fancy workout programming because muscles don't have cognitive abilities.

In reality, you will see better results if you don't keep changing your program and instead stick with the same exercises until you reach a plateau or have to switch exercises because you don't have the right equipment, don't have enough weight, are injured, etc.

Your muscles need time to perfect a specific movement before they can even call upon all the muscle fibers and coordinate them together.

If you were constantly switching exercises before you got the most out of an exercise, you wouldn't be building more muscle, but you would have to constantly restart your program before it got you the best results possible.

Also, excessive switching makes progressive overload difficult. You should aim for a steady increase in the amount of stress on your muscles instead of a completely new and shocking stress.

The best way to increase stress is by gradually increasing the weight you lift or the number of repetitions you do. This gives your body and muscles new but similar stimuli to adapt and respond to. The stress has to be similar or you won't make the correct progress.

Progressive overload should be used to measure whether your program is working and your body is improving, not as a way to shock and demolish your muscles.

So the point here is that for your muscles to keep growing in size and strength, they need to be challenged by progressive overload, not by changing exercises and your program.

EATING EXCESSIVE PROTEIN TO TRY TO BUILD MORE MUSCLE

Many gym-bros believe that if protein builds muscle, then chugging down more protein shakes means their bodies will be able to build more muscle.

There is a correlation between protein intake and muscle gain, but science doesn't support the claim that excessive protein consumption leads to more muscle.[17]

The amount of protein that research has proven beneficial for strength trainees ranges from 0.73 to 0.82 gram per pound (1.6 to 1.8 grams per kilogram) of your body weight.[18] The upper limit of 0.82 gram per pound per day (1.8 grams per kilogram per day) was given with a confidence interval and an extra margin of error (statistics-speak for "safety buffer") to ensure that all populations of people, even men whose bodies are capable of using an above-average protein intake, were definitely going to consume enough protein.

Anything above this doesn't translate to extra muscle. Many studies with varying populations have proven this.

For example, in many of the studies, researchers found that there was no difference in results in people who consumed twice to even three times as much protein as the standard recommendation.[19]

For those who grew up listening to old-school bodybuilders who insisted on eating 1 gram of protein per pound of body weight or 2.2 grams per kilogram, this recommendation may be difficult to accept.

This old-school guidance had no scientific proof to back it up, but it made for an easy recommendation, and when a person uses steroids, he needs to consume more protein.

So, more doesn't mean better; it just means more calories.[20]

Protein is also very filling, so it can make getting enough calories difficult if you're trying to bulk up. And prioritizing getting a lot of protein ahead of other essential nutrients can hurt your health and, in turn, your ability to build muscle.

DOING CIRCUIT TRAINING TO GET THE BEST OF BOTH WORLDS WHEN IT COMES TO BUILDING MUSCLE AND LOSING FAT

Circuit training is becoming more and more popular because it is believed to combine the muscle-building benefits of strength training with the fat-burning benefits of cardio.

In a typical strength-training program, you perform what are called "straight sets" of a single exercise.

Circuit training combines multiple back-to-back exercises into a single set, often by moving from one exercise to the next with little to no rest.

Circuit training may seem like it would have the same benefits as strength training and cardio because you move from one exercise to the next without stopping, but you also give your muscles time to rest before doing the same exercise again in the next set.

Unfortunately, since circuit training is so difficult, both neurologically and cardiovascularly, you will not be able to perform the same numbers of repetitions or use the same amounts of weight that you could if you took longer rest periods and caught your breath.

This results in less muscle growth, and because circuit training is so taxing, it causes more neuromuscular fatigue, worsens your technique and coordination, and is more likely to lead to injury.

As for fat loss, the science just doesn't support the idea that circuit training improves energy expenditure when compared with straight sets of strength training.

In one study, participants were put through a circuit-training session and a standard strength-training session. At the end of the study, the average difference in post-exercise energy expenditure (extra calories burned after finishing) between sessions was within 1 calorie.[21]

Another study comparing supersets (two exercises back-to-back) to standard strength-training sets showed that standard sets burned about 8 to 12 more calories during exercise, but grouped sets evened out the total calories burned post-exercise by burning about 6 to 8 more calories.[22]

Yet another study found that the increase in energy expenditure after an intense full-body circuit-training workout was a measly 18 calories more than with traditional sets.[23]

If you are willing to sacrifice muscle growth and are careful to perform each exercise with perfect technique, adding in circuit training can cut down on the time you spend working out and improve your cardiovascular endurance. Just don't expect it to be the best of both worlds.

◇◇◇

There you have it. Those are some of the top mistakes men make when it comes to building muscles.

More often than not, it comes down to trying to add enhancements to the pillars of muscle building or avoiding the tried-and-true methods due to misconceptions and misinformation.

Later in this book, we'll turn all this information into a simple, easy-to-use plan for changing your body. I'm hoping that you now understand what works and what doesn't, so creating a real-world diet and training program will be a walk in the park.

Once you're ready, flip to the next section, and let's go over the science behind leaning out and even getting to single-digit body fat levels to show off your newly developed muscles.

SECRET 3

–

THE SIMPLE SCIENCE
OF GETTING LEAN

CHAPTER 7

THE FOUR PILLARS OF WEIGHT CHANGE

This chapter is all about changing your weight in any direction you would like by building muscle, losing unwanted body fat, or both simultaneously.

It's easy to get confused about exactly what you need to do if you want to lose, gain, or maintain your weight. Fortunately, science has come surprisingly close to mathematically determining how to change body weight and total body composition.

The four fundamental pillars we are about to discuss will provide the structure for how to do it all using the most up-to-date research and science.

Unfortunately, this research is often misunderstood or misrepresented, leading to a lot of misinformation and mistakes.

So, before we begin, let me clear up some misconceptions.

First, science doesn't form an opinion. Instead, it presents facts (even if they are hard to accept) and lets you determine how you want to apply the information.

What you want to do with your weight is your business—your health, happiness, and mental well-being are most important. I'm just here to cut out the frustration of not getting the results you want and the confusion of not knowing what works and what doesn't.

Second, weight loss is not the same as fat loss; and weight gain doesn't equal fat gain. You can lose weight by going to the bathroom and gain weight by drinking a bottle of water.

These terms are often used interchangeably, such that when people talk about weight loss, they mean excess body fat loss, as though all weight lost is from only body fat. In reality, weight-loss diets often result in losing muscle mass and water weight, so you look lighter on the scale.

When I say "weight change," I mean either gaining muscle mass while minimizing fat gain, or decreasing your body fat percentage while maintaining or increasing your muscle mass.

Third, you need body fat to survive and function properly. Having a healthy amount of body fat (resulting in a healthy ratio of muscle mass to body fat) has been shown to improve health while lowering risks of preventable health issues and chronic conditions like heart attacks, strokes, diabetes, and even cancer.[1,2]

The problems arise when a person has too much or too little body fat, excessively eats unhealthy foods, and is not getting enough healthy nutrients.

Finally, losing unwanted body fat isn't as complicated as it's made out to be, and everyone can do it.

No one is naturally fat or genetically screwed so that they'll always be overweight. You can quickly shed unwanted body fat and maintain body fat levels that are healthy and that give you the body you've always wanted.

No matter the diet, fat loss and muscle gain will always come down to natural law and science, which I will outline in this chapter. Unfortunately, most people just miss the forest for the trees or try to do too much without first nailing down the basics.

PILLAR #1: ENERGY BALANCE

The concept of energy balance is based on the First Law of Thermodynamics, which states that energy in a system (in this case, the body) can only be used, transformed, or stored; it cannot be created or destroyed.

Energy balance is used to determine how your body mass changes over time based on how much energy you take in and how much energy you expend. In simple terms, we use it to regulate weight gain and loss.

An average person will expend energy through digestion, physical activity, and carrying out functions for survival and homeostasis. You must take in energy to keep your body functioning. Energy intake comes in the form of food and drinks you consume—in other words, your diet.

Some food components cannot be digested or broken down for energy and simply pass through you.

The energy that remains after digestion is metabolizable energy. This is energy that your body can use for different processes.

The amount of energy your diet contains and provides for your body is expressed as a number of calories. It's important to understand that a calorie is a measurement of energy, much like a gram is a measurement of weight. Specifically, and somewhat arbitrarily, a calorie is equal to the amount of energy needed to raise the temperature of 1 gram of water by 1 degree Celsius at a pressure of 1 atmosphere.

Technically, a nutritional calorie should be written with a capital C, or as a "kcal" (for *kilocalorie*). But nearly all of the nutritional field ignores this, so we'll stick with a lowercase c.

Scientists have been able to accurately determine the metabolizable energy content of food. These are the calorie numbers you see on nutrition labels, and the calories that allow us to accurately regulate fat loss or gain.

When you eat, your body either turns the food into energy you can use right away for movement, digestion, and other bodily functions, or stores the extra energy as body mass for later use.

You can use energy balance to manipulate your total body mass, including body fat levels, by adjusting your energy/calorie intake and energy/calorie expenditure. This means that if you lose energy from your body, you lose body mass too—and gaining extra energy from the food you eat equals gaining body mass.

If you keep track of your calorie intake, output, and weight change, you will realize three things:

- If you consume more calories than you burn, your body stores energy, and if you do it often enough, you gain weight.

- If you burn or expend more calories than you consume, your body loses energy, and when you do this often enough, you lose weight.

- If you take in the same number of calories as you expend, your body "breaks even" on energy, and when this happens consistently, you maintain your weight.

Here's how this process works: If you eat and drink more calories than you burn or expend, you create a positive energy balance, and your body stores a portion of the extra energy as either body fat or lean mass. And if you do this consistently, your body keeps storing the extra calories as body fat, resulting in weight gain.

However, if you consume fewer calories than you burn, you create a negative energy balance. This means that you've lost energy—but, for your body to stay alive and function, it requires a constant supply of energy. So your body turns to its stored energy to make up for the deficit and draw the energy it requires to keep functioning.

If you consistently eat fewer calories than you burn, your fat stores will slowly diminish, and you will become leaner. This is why all well-controlled research studies have come to the same conclusion: to lose weight, you need to expend more calories than you take in.

Now, in the average sedentary person who doesn't work out, body weight and total energy balance correlate strongly over the long term. They can use the simple math of body weight equaling calories in versus calories out.

But strength training turns all this on its head and shatters the idea that energy balance is equal to changes in your weight. This brings us to our next fat-loss pillar.

PILLAR #2: NUTRIENT PARTITIONING

When it comes to total body energy stored, lost, or maintained in your body, energy balance will always follow the First Law of Thermodynamics. You simply can't bend the laws of physics.

When looking at the overall mass of our bodies and the change in body mass, we will always go back to energy balance through calories consumed minus calories expended. Notice that I say "body mass" and "total body energy." This is because your body can maintain the same total energy but have a completely different composition and a different total body weight.

For example, you can maintain energy balance and change your total body weight by adjusting the amount of water your body is storing. However, our goal is not to just change your weight through adjusting your food to store or lose water weight. Our goal is to adjust the location where your body is storing energy and nutrients so that you completely change your body's composition to have more muscle and less fat.

For example, let's say you weigh 180 pounds and your body is composed of 55 pounds of fat mass (30% body fat) and 65 pounds of muscle mass. Your body has a lot of stored energy, primarily as fat mass.

But what if you kept the same amount of energy in your body but were able to rearrange it so that more of it was muscle mass and less was fat mass? You could still weigh 180 pounds, but you could instead have only 35 pounds of fat mass (20% body fat) and 85 pounds of muscle mass. Your body would be composed entirely differently because the location of nutrients and energy in your body would be more muscle and less fat.

This is because your body can store certain calories and nutrients in specific locations by breaking up the food you eat into smaller components and sending these components to different parts of your body based on where they are needed. This is known as nutrient partitioning—you partition (or split up) your nutrients and send them to different parts of your body where each specific nutrient is needed.

It is very important to understand this, because to lose body fat specifically, you need to:

- Increase the amount of energy you expend over the long term.

- Decrease the amount of energy you consume over the long term.

- Improve how your body partitions and uses nutrients.

The first two methods of losing body fat come down to energy balance, specifically calories in versus calories out, which we have already discussed. The third method, though, is where things start to change.

We will get into the other nutrients and how they help with nutrient partitioning in just a second, but for now, we are concerned with protein, building muscle, and how they relate to weight change and fat loss.

It is a much more difficult process for your body to build muscle than to create body fat, so your body preferentially stores extra calories as body fat if it doesn't need to build muscle mass. This is what happens to the average person who doesn't work out.

If, however, you present a large enough stimulus or stress, such as strength training, your body will "suck it up" and begin the energy-intensive process of building muscle.

This means that if your body has a good enough reason to create muscle versus body fat, it will take the food you eat, separate protein from everything else during digestion, and send it to be used for building muscles while the rest of your food is sent to different locations.

This ends up improving fat loss, because your body won't be breaking down protein into energy and turning that energy into body fat for later use. Instead, it will be creating muscle mass. You see, muscle is just a storage form of protein and energy.

Thanks to nutrient partitioning, you can create muscle while losing fat. And while your weight might not change on the scale (though it most likely will), your body will be losing fat and becoming denser and more amazing looking.

The same amount of energy will be either stored or burned, but it will be in different locations and will make up a different structure in your body.

Winning the game of nutrient partitioning is a matter of creating a calorie competition in which your fat tissues always lose and your muscle tissues always win. There are three methods for achieving this:

1. Increase muscle mass.

2. Decrease body fat levels.

3. Improve health markers.

Each of these three things poses a dilemma. One method will bolster the others, but you can't succeed with that first method until the others are improved.

However, when you apply all three of these methods slightly and simultaneously, each will enhance the others, which will set off a continuing cycle of improvements in all three.

Here is the improvement cycle: Decreased body fat level leads to improved health markers. Improved health markers mean better nutrient partitioning. Better nutrient partitioning means increased muscle-building potential. Increased muscle building and more muscle mass mean more calories burned in a day. More calories burned in a day equals the ability to eat more calories but still lose more fat. Less fat means . . .

And the cycle starts over. This time around, you're in a better starting position, so the cycle becomes more efficient.

In other words, the better your body gets at sending protein directly to protein synthesis, the more muscle you can build and the easier it is to lose fat. Also, building and maintaining muscles is very energy intensive, meaning it burns a lot of calories, which helps with fat loss.

Your body, through nutrient partitioning, can enhance muscle building and fat loss simultaneously.

Forget about the misconception that you can lose excess body fat only when you are in a calorie deficit and can gain muscle only when you are in a calorie surplus. This is simply not true.

Still, for this progress to happen, you must subject your body to the correct and sufficient stimuli, which you can get through strength training.

Along with strength training, your body needs to be as healthy as possible and well fed with proper nutrition in order to partition nutrients in the best way possible, increase your fat loss, and maximize your muscle building. This brings us to our next pillar of weight change.

PILLAR #3: MACRONUTRIENT METABOLISM

Are certain calories more fattening than others? Does the type of carbs matter when it comes to fat loss? Does eating fat make you fat? Does consuming more fat mean that your body becomes better at burning fat, leading to more body fat lost? Is sugar bad for you?

If we look at the different sources (food and drinks) from which you can get your calories, weight change becomes a bit different—and there is a lot of misinformation out there.

Your diet supplies your body with energy and nutrients. The nutrients you take in are generally separated into two categories based on their functions in your body and how much of them you consume. They are:

- Macronutrients

- Micronutrients

Macronutrients are bigger molecules that are eaten in larger amounts and can be broken down to be used for energy. The three chemical structures of macronutrients that we care about are proteins, carbohydrates, and fats.

Micronutrients are consumed in much smaller amounts (*micro-* means "small"). These are the vitamins and minerals, which are necessary for your health and help your body perform most of its functions.

When you consume proteins, carbohydrates, and fats, your digestive system breaks them down into substrates that can be transported throughout your body and used in various ways. Substrates are the different sources of nutrients and energy your body requires to perform daily activities and maintain its functions. They are the bare essentials that your body can actually use.

For instance, proteins are catabolized to their substrate of amino acids, carbohydrates are mainly broken down into glucose, and fats are primarily broken down into fatty acids.

At any given time during the day, your body is breaking down, or metabolizing, its own stored substrates, like body fat and glycogen, along with macronutrients from your diet. It then sends the substrates to different parts of your body to keep your brain functioning, build muscle, complete your daily activities, repair and rebuild tissues, and more.

In fact, your body is most likely breaking down and building fat as well as muscle mass at this very moment. Thanks to nutrient partitioning, your body can perform both of these processes separately but at the same time.

However, if you didn't eat all three macronutrients in your diet, your body wouldn't be able to complete these tasks, let alone function properly.

Your body uses different substrates from each macronutrient for completing different functions; each offers different health benefits, and all three macronutrients are needed to ensure a balance of necessary nutrients.

When your body is healthy, getting the proper nutrients, and able to do all of its necessary functions well, it can optimally partition nutrients to build muscle, which, as we just talked about in the last pillar, helps you lose fat.

But if your body is unhealthy, it will have more pressing matters to attend to and will send nutrients somewhere else before building muscle, because building muscle takes a lot of energy.

For example, if you are infected with a disease, your body won't waste energy trying to get you jacked. Instead, it will do everything in its power to fight that disease.

So, by feeding your body the correct proteins, carbohydrates, and dietary fats, you can improve your health, help your body function optimally, improve nutrient partitioning, ramp up the amount of muscle you can build, and increase the rate at which you lose body fat.

Having said that, there are also two other ways that macronutrient metabolism can improve your fat loss.

When it comes to fat loss, research has pinpointed three mechanisms by which including a specific macronutrient and substrate in your diet can tip the scales.[3] These mechanisms are:

1. Increasing muscle growth

2. Increasing metabolic rate during digestion

3. Reducing hunger (creating satiety)

If a macronutrient substrate can help with at least one of these three things, then it can help improve fat loss. The goal is to increase the calories you burn or reduce the calories you eat by simply eating more of the correct nutrients.

Once you know which macronutrient substrate can help with fat loss, you can add foods that contain it into your meal plan—which we will cover in an upcoming section. To achieve this, you need proper knowledge of the macronutrients and their effects on your health and body.

Macronutrient #1: Proteins

Protein has many more roles than simply helping you build muscle. However, protein intake becomes even more essential when you're working out regularly, because it helps meet your body's amino acid demands for repair, recovery, and building.

By now, you should know that getting enough of each amino acid by eating enough protein every day is essential for your health and physique. When it comes to fat loss, a high-protein diet can help with all three of the fat-loss mechanisms discussed above, making it an ideal dieting strategy for fat loss.

First, a high protein intake can lead to more muscle growth. Muscle growth is a very energy-intensive process, requiring your body to tap into a lot of extra energy that typically wouldn't be used if you didn't consume that much protein, or at least enough protein to build muscle.

Along with the energy it takes to build muscle, the more muscle you have, the more calories your body burns daily.[4] This makes you expend more energy daily, which can help you lose fat or keep you from gaining fat.

Second, your body needs to use calories and energy to digest the food you eat. Scientifically, this is called the thermic effect of food, or TEF.

To break down protein, your body burns more calories than when it metabolizes carbs and fats. Again, this leads to a higher daily energy expenditure, which can help you lose fat or keep you from gaining it.

Finally, as the most satiating macronutrient, protein makes you feel fuller and stay fuller longer. This means you're less likely to feel hungry throughout the day, which makes you eat less—and eating less can lead to less body fat.

But protein is not a magical macronutrient that goes against the laws of nature and thermodynamics.

Protein contains calories—4 calories per gram, to be exact—and will always follow the law of energy balance. Protein can be turned into fat or used as energy when your body and muscles have enough amino acids to do what they need to do or when you don't get enough energy from other sources.

So, if you want to torch more fat and build more muscle, you will want to be on a high-protein, calorie-deficit diet.

Macronutrient #2: Carbohydrates

Carbs often get a bad rap, especially regarding weight gain, because carbs are composed of sugars. Most people equate eating carbs with gaining excess fat, but in a real sense, carbs aren't as bad as people make them sound—and *sugar* is a buzzword.

In fact, once you understand how carbs are composed and function in your body, it is easier to see how they can be an ally in your health, fat loss, and muscle-gaining goals.

There are two major categories of carbohydrates:

1. Simple carbohydrates

2. Complex carbohydrates

Simple carbohydrates have one or two sugar molecules and are further divided into monosaccharides and disaccharides. The term *monosaccharide* simply means "one sugar." Disaccharides are composed of two monosaccharides. *Mono-* for "one," *di-* for "two," and *saccharide* for "sugar."

Complex carbohydrates have three or more sugar molecules. The two forms of complex carbohydrates are oligosaccharides and polysaccharides.

Both are made up of a long chain of monosaccharides linked together. Oligosaccharides have approximately 3 to 10 monosaccharides combined together, and polysaccharides are a long chain of 11 to 1,000 or more sugar molecules.

All carbohydrates, no matter what food or drink they come from, are broken down by your body into one of three things: glucose, fructose, or fiber. Most carbohydrates are broken down into glucose or fructose, which is then slowly released into the bloodstream and used or stored in different parts of your body. The only time this doesn't happen is when a carb contains dietary fibers, which are only partly digestible.

The major difference in digestion between complex and simple carbs is the rate at which they are broken down. Due to their chemical structures, simple carbs tend to be broken down into glucose faster than complex carbs. Complex carbs have more combined sugar molecules and are often more complex molecular structures, so they just take longer to break down.

It's like pulling apart a structure of Legos one at a time. If only two Legos are stuck together, you can quickly separate them into individual pieces. But if there are many pieces, a poly-Lego structure if you will, then it will take more time to break down into single Lego pieces.

When it comes to body-weight change, your body doesn't care whether a carb is simple or complex. It only cares about the number of calories consumed, not where they come from. So, a carb is a carb because it has calories—4 calories per gram, just like protein.

Instead of focusing on simple versus complex carbs, you should concentrate on what nutrients the carbohydrate source contains.

Just like with protein, a macronutrient's ability to improve fat loss comes down to how filling the food is (satiety), whether the food improves muscle growth through anabolism or improves health, and whether it burns extra calories during digestion.

The reason why most people, including nutritionists and even doctors, associate simple carbo-hydrates with weight gain is that foods with added sugar are often more delectable, less filling, and composed of fewer nutrients per calorie. This is referred to as being calorie-dense. When food is calorie-dense, tastes delicious, and doesn't make you feel full (the trifecta for weight gain), you will often consume more of it, quickly increasing your calorie intake.

The carbohydrate sources that can help with fat loss are often the opposite and are referred to as nutrient-dense. Specifically, they contain dietary fibers, vitamins, and minerals.

This is where carbohydrates really shine when it comes to health and fat loss.

Dietary fibers, which are found in some complex carbohydrates, are very satiating. This means they make you feel fuller longer, which can help keep you from overeating.

Plus, fiber has many health benefits, including improving gut health and helping to reduce your risk of cancer.[5]

Also, if there is one thing that all respected nutrition experts can agree on when it comes to eating carbs, it's that fruits and vegetables are a must.[6] Not only do they have fiber, but they also contain vitamins and minerals your body needs. Taking in a variety of fruits and vegetables can improve your health markers, inflammation levels, psychological well-being, and, in turn, nutrient partitioning.[7]

So, eating specific carbs can improve your health, leading to better nutrient partitioning and muscle-building potential.

As a final benefit, your body will burn more calories than usual while digesting fibrous carbohydrates.

As you can see, eating certain carbs can help you efficiently lose weight by improving how your body partitions nutrients, increasing your muscle-building potential, burning more calories during digestion, and making you feel less hungry after a meal.

Macronutrient #3: Dietary Fats

Dietary fats (the fats we eat) are mostly made up of three things: triglycerides, phospholipids (which are part of cell membranes), and cholesterol.

Triglycerides make up 95% of the fat that we eat. So, when we talk about fat in nutrition, we usually mean triglycerides, and more specifically, fatty acids, which are their main components. Triglycerides are made up of three fatty acids attached to a glycerol backbone, which is how they got their name.

Fatty acids are used throughout the body for different health processes, providing structure for cell membranes, and giving your cells energy.

When used for energy production, fatty acids provide 9 calories per gram. This makes them much more energy-dense than carbohydrates and proteins.

However, that doesn't mean that taking in triglycerides leads to more body fat, because dietary fat isn't the same as body fat, and it doesn't convert directly into body fat. It also doesn't mean that "going keto" (eating a very high-fat diet) is the key to endless energy, better brain functioning, and burning more "fat." It will all come down to your total energy balance.

When used as a nutrient, fatty acids are vital for your body to function correctly because they have many health benefits, such as:

- Aiding in the absorption of vitamins A, D, E, and K.

- Supporting hormone development.

- Promoting healthy hair and skin.

The different functions that a fatty acid will serve are based on whether the fatty acid is completely saturated with hydrogen atoms or unsaturated due to missing at least one hydrogen atom.

The three types of fatty acids you consume in your diet and need to know about for health, muscle growth, and fat loss are:

- Saturated fatty acids (fully saturated with hydrogen atoms).

- Monounsaturated fatty acids (having one double-bonded carbon).

- Polyunsaturated fatty acids (having two or more double-bonded carbons).

Just like the other two macronutrients we've looked at, dietary fats can help with body fat loss if they can help you build muscle and improve nutrient partitioning, increase calories burned through digestion, or reduce your feelings of hunger.

Out of the three fat-loss mechanisms, dietary fats are the most beneficial for promoting muscle growth. This is because of their positive effects on hormone production, and certain fatty acids even have other anabolic properties.

In particular, saturated fatty acids are the building blocks for cholesterol, which your body needs to make certain anabolic and sex hormones. So, when combined with strength training, consuming a little bit more cholesterol might help create more muscle and lead to less body fat.[8]

In fact, fatty acids have been shown to positively influence your body's testosterone levels, which can substantially increase your muscle-building ability.[9,10]

Multiple research studies have shown that when dietary fat intake was increased from about 20% to 40% of total daily energy intake, the anabolic hormones testosterone, growth hormone, and IGF-1 increased by approximately 20%.[11,12]

So, a higher-fat diet may improve your overall body composition and muscle-building potential by increasing your testosterone levels and improving other anabolic hormone production.[13,14]

Along with saturated fatty acids, both of the unsaturated fatty acids, monounsaturated and poly-unsaturated, have been shown to be beneficial for overall health, increasing lean body mass and reducing fat mass.[15,16]

Some polyunsaturated fatty acids are even categorized as "essential fatty acids" because our bodies cannot produce them. This means we have to get them from food or supplements to prevent poor health and even early death.

However, the two most important fatty acids are omega-3 fatty acids and omega-6 fatty acids. Omega-3 and omega-6 fatty acids are made from certain essential fatty acids or can be consumed on their own through your diet and supplementation.

Omega-3s have the amazing potential benefit of stepping up the rate at which your body synthesizes (creates) protein.[17] Enhanced protein synthesis increases lean body mass through muscle growth and a faster metabolism, which can increase fat loss.[18,19]

Here are some of the other health benefits that omega-3 fatty acids bestow on your body:

- Decreased inflammation[20]

- Reduced depression and improved mood through lower cortisol levels[21]

- Protection against excessive muscle damage if you are strength training; hence muscle growth[22]

- Increased production of testosterone[23]

- Faster body fat loss[24]

- Improved cognitive performance

- Better insulin sensitivity[25]

- Protection for joints

Omega-6s, the other important essential fatty acids, are much more common in the average diet. Research conducted on omega-6 fatty acids shows that they lower the risk of heart disease, which is a huge win for your health.[26]

In general, you should try to get all the fatty acids in your diet, with special consideration to omega-3s, because they all help your body make hormones, keep you healthy, and help you lose fat.

PILLAR #4: SUSTAINABILITY

Throughout this chapter, I have said that you need to do everything over the long term to get results. Changing your body's composition is a long-term process, but it's an amazing one. It is one of the few endeavors in life where you can noticeably see and feel the differences every single day.

Too many people chase rapid results, try to use pure willpower, or stick to bad diets in the pursuit of body-weight change. Unfortunately, even if it works for a little while, this will always lead to diet failure and poor results.

Consistency and adherence are the keys to truly changing your weight, losing fat, and gaining muscle. None of these can be done without ensuring that your diet, meal plan, nutrition program, or whatever you want to call it is sustainable for the long term.

The best diets aren't diets; they are lifestyle changes that prioritize exercise and healthy eating. They are simple, include the foods you enjoy, are based on your life and food availability, and still get results.

Sustainable dieting becomes a routine that allows you to put most of your life on autopilot so you can concentrate on what matters most to you (outside of your health).

All three pillars before this are worthless if you can only stick to your strength-training and nutrition programs for a week.

Instead, find a way to eat your ideal number of calories and nutrients that you can stick with. It's all about you and finding what helps you sustain your efforts and turn dieting into a healthy long-term lifestyle. Then you simply make consistent incremental adjustments to reach your weight-change and muscle-building goals. Incremental action compounds for better, easier, and more efficient results.

In later sections, you will learn how to create a sustainable, enjoyable, and results-driven nutrition program.

◇◇◇

Scientifically speaking, changing your weight is pretty straightforward. You eat the correct number of calories based on how many calories you expend in a day and whether you want to lose fat or increase your total body mass.

If these calories come from certain food sources, you can provide your body with the correct nutrients to build muscle, lose fat, and improve your health simultaneously.

This might change your body weight, but it will most definitely change your body composition. When all of it is done simultaneously, it is referred to as body recomposition, or just recomping.

Not only is it possible to build muscle and lose fat at the same time, but body recomposition should almost always be the goal and the result of your diet.

This doesn't matter if your diet is so bland and strict that you can't maintain it and consistently adhere to its requirements. Creating a sustainable diet is where physiology, psychology, and implementation intertwine into real-world results.

In upcoming sections, we'll apply these four pillars to create an optimized nutrition program for fast-tracking your fat-loss and muscle-building efforts.

CHAPTER 8

THE MOST COMMON MISTAKES AND MISCONCEPTIONS THAT HALT MEN'S FAT LOSS

When most people decide to embark on a weight-loss journey, they look for advice on how to do it by either digging through the Internet or asking friends and family around them. The advice they end up with promises to help them shed excess body fat as quickly as possible because their friend has found what works for them, or there's been some "new study" done that content creators or fitness and nutrition companies embellish to sell a product or stay relevant.

And since we all love seeing immediate results, most of us end up victims of lies and misinformation. Unfortunately, losing unwanted body fat is not something that happens overnight. For the most part, it takes smart choices and lots of patience to lose weight.

With all the conflicting information available, it can be tough to separate fact from fiction. So I'm about to take aim at some of the most common mistakes men make regarding weight loss.

These mistakes are often the result of big myths and misconceptions and may keep you from making real progress and prevent you from being healthy. Learn from these mistakes, or history is doomed to repeat itself.

BELIEVING THAT YOU ARE GENETICALLY FAT AND CAN'T LOSE WEIGHT

When people believe that it's impossible to lose weight due to a factor that is out of their control, such as genetics, they will put in less effort, even if it is subconscious. After all, what's the point of trying to eat healthily and look great if it's genetically impossible for you to succeed?

People who are overweight because of bad eating habits and inaccurate calorie counting will have a harder time losing weight and building muscle. This is because chronic inflammation, poor carbo-hydrate tolerance, and hormone imbalances lead to poor nutrient processing, fewer calories burned digesting food, more fat storage, and less muscle creation.[1,2]

However, there is no such thing as a genetic body fat percentage or level of fat mass that your body is predisposed to always maintain. Even recent research proves that there is no "body fat set point" that can never be altered.[3]

In reality, most people can't lose weight because they're consuming more calories than they burn over time.

If you follow closely, you will find that people who claim to have a specific genetic body-fat set point actually take in a lot more calories than they burn. This is because most people simply don't know how to estimate the actual number of calories they consume.

You might be gaining weight not because of your genes, but because you can't accurately determine how many calories you're eating. The calories you consume matter a lot when it comes to weight management, and underestimating or overestimating affects your body differently.

It's very easy to screw up your calories because the number of calories indicated on a food package or given on a restaurant menu is often inaccurate, and people who stick to preparing and cooking their own food often mismeasure their foods. Unfortunately, many people don't realize this and are left feeling genetically screwed.

ACTIVELY AVOIDING COUNTING CALORIES

No one wants to be told they need to exercise more and eat less. They want an easier and faster way to get the job done that doesn't require them to change or admit that they were wrong.

Nonetheless, science and research have been able to disprove every hypothesis as to why energy balance may be incorrect. In fact, many studies and meta-analyses have shown that calorie counting is the most effective tactic to help people lose excess body fat.[4,5] The most recent studies also show that weight-loss programs incorporating calorie counting are the most effective.[6,7] This is because counting calories helps you keep track of what you're consuming so that you don't over- or undereat.[8]

Calorie counting is so effective at ensuring results that professional bodybuilders looking to drop to incredibly low body fat percentages for competitions count their calories precisely.

The confusion often comes from not understanding how calories work in your body and how all the studies accurately measure energy balance. The studies place people in metabolic wards to precisely measure every single calorie. Then researchers adjust each variable that might affect a person's calorie expenditure, such as the thermic effect of food (TEF), total fat-free body mass, non-exercise activity thermogenesis (NEAT), and more, to ensure that they can determine precisely how accurate calorie counting is and create equations for us to calculate our energy expenditure accurately.

Sure, the science can get confusing, but tracking your calories both in and out is the best method of ensuring consistent results. It may be challenging to do at times, but the science doesn't lie.

Keeping tabs on what you eat and the results you get will keep you on track, help you concentrate on your goals, and allow you to make minor adjustments to get even better results. So, when in doubt, count calories.

TRYING TO TARGET THE EXACT LOCATION WHERE YOU WANT TO LOSE FAT

I'm sure you've come across "the five moves you need to do to build a six-pack" or "a 6-minute core workout for burning belly fat" and possibly even seen advertisements to "drop stubborn fat around your waist with a hormonal reset."

Unfortunately, you can create the perfect environment for fat loss through diet and exercise, do as many crunches and sit-ups as you want, or buy expensive supplements, and still, you'll never be able to lose only belly fat, because fat loss occurs in a whole-body fashion.

The muscles or areas of your body you're training don't matter, because your body fat is broken down and transported through your blood to where it needs to go to be used for energy or nutrients. Then your body stores any excess energy as body fat in the same location the other body fat just left, i.e., your adipose tissue.

Muscle growth occurs in the muscles that are trained, so growing specific muscles can make it appear that you are losing fat in that area, but you are just spreading out the same body fat over a greater surface area.

This is similar to the pseudoscience that says that you can rearrange your body fat by "fixing" your hormones. In reality, your body fat storage locations are heavily based on your genetics, with your age and ethnicity also having a small effect.[9] Hormones actually play a minuscule part in the location of fat storage from person to person. However, poor hormonal health from being unhealthy and overweight can significantly affect muscle growth and total body fat levels.[10]

Higher testosterone levels lead to more fat storage around a person's waist, while higher estrogen levels promote fat storage around the hips and thighs. This is often touted as the classic apple body shape for men and pear body shape for women. But these body shapes are caused mainly by your male or female genetics, not by your hormones.

Your male genetics outweigh (pun intended) the body fat spot reduction that might come from taking a supplement to slightly adjust your testosterone, insulin, estrogen, IGF-1, and other hormone levels. It would take a steroid level of hormones to trump where you genetically store body fat.

CUTTING CARBS FROM YOUR DIET BECAUSE SUGARS WILL MAKE YOU FAT

Is a calorie a calorie when it comes to the type of carbohydrate you eat?

This topic can get really complicated and overly scientific, so instead, let's look at what science has proven through multiple research studies comparing simple carbs, like straight table sugar, and diets made up of complex, "healthy" carbs.

In a six-month study with 390 participants, half of the group ate a diet high in complex carbs, and the other half ate a diet high in simple carbs. Both diets had the exact same amount of total carbohydrates and the same number of calories.

At the end of the six months, there were no differences in fat loss or muscle retention. And participants' blood lipids (fat in the blood) were similar.[11]

Researchers did another study that replaced part of a diet's complex carbs with simple carbs to determine body-composition changes.[12] At the end of the study, there was no difference in body composition. This means that muscle mass and fat mass remained the same when protein, fats, and calories remained the same.

In the end, research has proven over and over again that for fat loss, it doesn't matter if the carb is simple or complex as long as the total calories from the carbs remain the same.

The major problem that most nutrition experts have with sugar and added sugars is that they increase your calorie intake but don't fill you up, and they make meals more palatable. Basically, sugar-laden foods taste delicious but don't reduce your hunger. That's a recipe for excess calorie consumption and weight gain.

To back this up, many studies show that consuming diets with different amounts of sugars but the same number of total calories results in no change in body weight.[13,14,15]

CUTTING CARBS AND EATING MORE DIETARY FAT TO TURN YOUR BODY INTO A "FAT-BURNING MACHINE"

Looking at cutting carbs from a different perspective, can ditching carbs in place of a high-fat diet, like the popular Atkins and ketogenic diets, turn your body into a lean, mean, fat-burning machine?

Unfortunately, high-fat-diet worshippers often miss the forest for the trees. High-fat diets can be beneficial when done correctly, but the assumption that this will lead to less body fat than other diets is wrong.

Your body is constantly in flux. If we just look at body fat by itself, your body is continually building new body fat and breaking down current body fat. When you eat, your body breaks down your food and stores a lot of energy as body fat to be used later. Once this process is finished, your body will use that stored energy to survive and complete different functions for the rest of the day. This process occurs repeatedly throughout the day based on your meals and activities.

If you looked at a snapshot in time of your body's composition, you would only see whether your body was burning body fat for energy or storing body fat to be used later. You could be consistently losing body fat day to day, but if you looked at what your body was doing directly after a meal, you would think you were gaining weight due to all the body fat being created.

So it's not about the substrate that you are currently metabolizing for energy (in this example, that would be fatty acids); it's about your energy balance over the long term that will dictate how your body fat changes.

So, it would be best if you didn't ditch carbs entirely. In fact, completely cutting out carbs from your diet can make losing fat more difficult due to less fiber, vitamins, minerals, and phytonutrients, and a less sustainable and enjoyable diet.

CUTTING FATS FROM YOUR DIET BECAUSE THEY EASILY TURN INTO BODY FAT

Just because dietary fat has the word *fat* in it doesn't mean it makes you become what you eat.

Dietary fat is not turned directly into body fat. Instead, it is first broken down to be used as energy or fuel for your cells or other essential body functions.

It may be easier for your body to store dietary fat as body fat in the sense that it is a more direct conversion, but it isn't easier energy-wise for your body to do this, which is what really matters for your body.

Also, dietary fats might have over twice as many calories per gram as proteins and carbs, but unless this leads to excess energy intake, the number of calories of fat you eat compared to calories of carbs or protein doesn't matter.

Your body can't store excess energy if it doesn't exist.

This higher number only makes fat more calorically dense, but what matters for weight gain or loss is the total calories consumed versus those burned, no matter where they come from.

Many studies have proven that the ratio of fats in your diet doesn't matter; what matters most is the total number of calories.[16,17,18,19]

Research also shows that healthy fats can speed up your metabolism and help you lose weight by increasing your protein synthesis rates and building more lean body mass.[20,21]

You need to eat dietary fat to have a healthy diet. Fats help build cells, aid in the absorption of certain vitamins, and much more. Unsaturated fats, like fish oil, avocados, and nuts, help boost brain and skin health and even fuel weight loss.

AVOIDING HIGH-CARB DIETS BECAUSE THEY LEAD TO MORE OF YOUR FOOD BEING STORED AS BODY FAT

This myth continues with the thought that if you consume a lot of carbs, your body will store more dietary fat as body fat since it doesn't need the fat for energy.

Your body's use of fatty acids for energy highly depends on the amount of carbohydrates you consume because your body prefers to use carbohydrates for energy. If you eat a lot of carbs, your cells become glucose-rich, and your body will store more of the fat you eat (along with any excess glucose and amino acids) instead of using it for immediate energy. Enough immediately available energy will always stimulate the creation and storage of body fat.

However, in a fasted state hours after a meal, your body needs a way to keep fueling your metabolic processes. This leads to an acceleration in body fat breakdown to fuel your activities and keep you alive. In the end, the amount of energy stored as body fat after a meal will balance itself out by being used for energy when all your food is digested.

Think of it like a bank. When you want to take money out of your account, you don't get the same $20 bill you put in last week. Instead, you get a different $20 bill, and $20 is deducted from your account. At one time your balance was higher, but over time you broke even.

NOT CUTTING ENOUGH CALORIES IN FEAR OF DAMAGING YOUR METABOLISM AND SWITCHING YOUR BODY INTO "STARVATION MODE"

When you start to get leaner and your calorie intake starts to decrease, your metabolism also decreases. Most of the time, this is simply because you are eating fewer calories, so you are burning fewer calories through digestion, and because you are losing mass from your body, which reduces the number of calories you burn for survival.

However, your metabolism actually decreases faster than you would expect based on the two reasons mentioned above.

This is called "starvation mode" because your body works to become more efficient and burn fewer calories than usual. This is done to keep you from starving and to conserve energy for the unknown future. Scientifically, this is known as adaptive thermogenesis.

Starvation mode sounds scary, but your body will often slow your metabolism by only about 10% of your basal metabolic rate. This equates to only about 100 to 300 fewer calories burned per day.

Your body does this by making your movements throughout the day more efficient and cutting back on spontaneous activity, like fidgeting and bobbing your head.

Plus, all this is based on your body fat percentage, not on the number of calories you eat.[22]

So eating fewer calories might have the placebo effect of making you feel like you have less energy, but starvation mode doesn't begin until you reach around 10% body fat.

In fact, research has shown that fast weight loss doesn't slow your metabolism more than slow weight loss.[23]

Your metabolic rate is based on your body composition at the time. So, your metabolism will change as your body changes.

Your metabolism doesn't permanently stay "damaged" from dieting.[24] If you gain the weight back, your body will ratchet up your metabolism by a similar percentage.

To back this up, a review was done on extreme weight-loss scenarios, such as anorexic women, bodybuilders during contest prep, malnourished individuals, wrestlers aggressively cutting weight for a competition, and more. The study found no evidence of metabolic damage. Zero.[25]

PRIORITIZING CARDIO OVER STRENGTH TRAINING FOR WEIGHT LOSS

A large-scale meta-analysis of more than 200 professional studies looking at long-term fat loss in general populations found that strength training is better for losing body fat than cardio or a combination of strength training and cardio.[26]

The misconception that you need to do cardio training with your strength training to get lean implies that one form of exercise is better for losing weight and the other is better for gaining weight—that they are mutually exclusive without any overlap.

Except we've already talked about how, when you do strength training, nutrient partitioning lets you build muscle and lose fat at the same time. In reality, strength training shares the same benefit that cardio has when it comes to fat loss: it burns calories. Research shows that cardio and strength training both burn about a few hundred to 600 calories per hour depending on intensity, experience, and body weight.[27]

However, strength training has a benefit that cardio training doesn't: it builds muscle, which is a very energy-intensive process.

Plus, the more muscle mass you have, the more calories your body burns daily.[28]

So, when it comes to the total number of calories burned over time, strength training blows cardio out of the water.

Keep in mind, though, that this places heavy emphasis on the "calories out" part of the energy balance equation while neglecting the "calories in" side of the equation, which is a recipe for disaster.

In fact, exercise is not more effective for fat loss than simply eating equivalently fewer calories.[29]

Luckily, when done at a higher intensity, cardio and strength training are very appetite-suppressing.[30] If you are training hard, your body is too busy trying to survive to worry about eating.

However, strength training has been found to be even more appetite-suppressing than cardio, leading to fewer calories eaten post-exercise and to fat loss in the long term.[31]

Unfortunately for cardio devotees, once your cardio session is over, your body will conserve energy and burn fewer calories than usual for the rest of the day.[32] So you might have less appetite, but you will also engage in less movement throughout the day, thanks to slower and more efficient movements, less fidgeting, and more.

Strength training, surprisingly, doesn't suffer from this problem.[33]

Finally, cardio is often very difficult to adhere to unless you enjoy going on bike rides, jogging, taking long walks, etc. Eventually, most people fall off the wagon due to any number of factors.

In fact, a 2011 meta-analysis that reviewed 14 highly controlled studies with over 1,840 participants showed that cardio was ineffective at achieving weight loss in overweight individuals. After 6 months of doing cardio, participants had lost only about 3.5 pounds (1.6 kilograms) on average and only 3.75 pounds (1.7 kilograms) after 12 months.[34]

While strength training can suffer from the same problems, most people find it much more sustainable, which is a huge but often overlooked benefit for fat loss.

The science and research speak for themselves: strength training isn't just for building muscles; it is also better for fat loss.

EATING SMALLER AMOUNTS OF FOOD FREQUENTLY INSTEAD OF FEWER, LARGER MEALS

When you eat, your body uses energy to digest your food. As mentioned earlier, the energy needed to break down and digest specific foods is called the thermic effect of food, or TEF.

Eating frequent small meals is often touted as a great strategy to keep your metabolism revved up all day, burn more calories by digesting food more frequently, stave off hunger, and, in turn, lose weight. But this theory disintegrates when you compare the length of digestion, the total number of calories burned, and the sustainability of this dieting strategy.

The uptick in metabolism and calories burned during digestion of smaller meals is small but happens more often, while the increase caused by larger meals lasts much longer but happens less often.

When all's said and done, the number of calories burned during digestion evens out. So, there is no (or very, very minimal) difference in fat loss between the two eating strategies.

Researchers actually debunked this myth about the benefit of frequent, smaller meals over 40 years ago. In a 1982 study, researchers compared the effects of meal frequency on energy expenditure. Two groups were given the same macronutrient and energy content, but one group was fed two meals and the other group had six meals.

In the end, the total energy expenditure was the same for the two groups.[35] And all subsequent studies have shown the same.

Plus, having to determine the number of calories and macronutrients in each meal to prevent accidental overeating and unaccounted-for snacking; having to create five or six meals every day; and finding the time to eat those meals is very difficult for most people to adhere to. It's a nightmare just to plan your meals so they don't get in the way of your work, social life, or training.

Overall, eating fewer but larger meals has been shown to be more effective for weight loss.

BEING UNNECESSARILY RESTRICTIVE BY CUTTING SPECIFIC FOODS (GLUTEN, DAIRY, BREAD, RED MEAT, ETC.) COMPLETELY OUT OF YOUR DIET

Every year there is a new scapegoat food that is to blame for why you can't lose weight.

A few buzzwords are thrown around, and the next thing you know, you think you have celiac disease because you sometimes get bloated when eating wheat, you need to avoid dairy because you are finally convinced that human bodies aren't meant to drink cow's milk, or you need to stay away from foods that you might naturally eat more of and overconsume.

This diet strategy plays to the hypochondriac in everyone, creates a very restrictive diet, produces a placebo effect, and leads to poor mental health when you eventually fail to keep cutting that food out of your diet.

It works like this: You think that if you don't eat X, you will lose weight and feel better. You believe you will feel better, so you convince yourself that you do feel better. You also eat fewer foods that are often overconsumed, so you lose weight.

For example, if you avoid gluten, you will usually lower your intake of bread, pasta, and baked goods. Likewise, if you avoid dairy, you won't eat cheese, cream cheese, ice cream, pizza, yogurt, and so on.

Now, all you have to do is completely avoid a particular food source for the rest of your life. (Good luck with that.)

As you should know by now, no single food will make you fat, and cutting food X will not lead to more or less weight loss, because it always comes down to calories in versus calories out.

However, I need to note that this pertains only to cutting out foods for fat loss. There are foods that are considered unhealthy, even carcinogenic (cancer-causing), and if you do have celiac disease or are lactose intolerant, then your body really does process these foods differently.

◇◇◇

If you've ever tried to lose weight, I'm sure you've heard of many people making these same mistakes. And I'm sure you've even made some of them yourself in the past. I've been there, so I understand.

You must stop believing them now if you want to progress in your fitness journey. Following these myths will make your journey much more difficult as you start to set up your meal plan and work toward your dream body.

These misguided tactics will make your diet very restrictive and hard to stick to. They can cause excess psychological stress through worrying whether you're doing everything correctly. They can waste your time and effort with little to show for it, and even lead to an unhealthy lifestyle and diet.

Instead, in an upcoming section, we will examine the pillars of fat loss and what has been proven to work in the real world with real men while producing the best results possible in the shortest amount of time, and we'll create an enjoyable meal plan that includes your favorite foods, demolishes hunger, builds muscle, and sheds fat.

PART III

THE PROGRAM VARIABLES

SECRET 4

-

EVERYTHING YOU NEED TO CREATE AN EFFECTIVE NUTRITION PROGRAM

CHAPTER 9

YOUR ONLY FOUR GUIDELINES FOR EFFECTIVE DIETING

Dieting can be very difficult, but it doesn't need to be. In fact, to truly succeed at dieting in the context of building an impressive body, dieting should be simple.

It shouldn't require much effort or willpower and should rarely become unpleasant. Facing constant hunger or forcing yourself to be strict and eat bland foods is a clear sign that your current diet isn't working for you.

Your diet is failing you, which will lead to diet failure.

To remedy this, you should follow a diet that's structured and balanced yet allows for flexibility. Pair this with a flexible dieting mindset, where you don't need to be exact and every misstep is just a learning experience, and you'll get better results over the long term.

The beauty of this flexible dieting approach is that it has only four simple guidelines and follows a dieting hierarchy.

Every other diet fad or method is just a drop in the bucket compared to these four things. So, if you can remember these four guidelines and always resort back to them, you'll be golden.

Flexible dieting also has a straightforward hierarchy of variables. This hierarchy is based on the order of importance of the different variables used when creating a meal plan, which variables will give you the most results, and which ones should take up more of your concentration.

The chapters in this section follow this variable hierarchy. You start by determining calories, then split those calories into macronutrients, split those macronutrients into food sources, and finally, time your nutrients.

THE FOUR DIETING GUIDELINES

You'll follow the four guidelines below to create a nutrition program that helps you efficiently build an amazing physique.

Each guideline is intertwined with the other three to work together for better and easier results. So, it's important to follow each one to get the best results with the least amount of work.

The four guidelines are:

1. Balance goals and reality.

2. Eat for weight change.

3. Eat to build muscle.

4. Improve diet quality.

When creating your meal plan in this section and upcoming ones, you will draw on each of these precepts in one manner or another. If you wander outside these guidelines, your diet will become immensely more difficult.

Guideline #1: Balance Goals and Reality

Nutrition for building muscle and getting lean follows pillars of science and research that provide the foundation for creating a meal plan.

In a lab and with perfect willpower, you could implement each of these, draw up the perfect meal plan, and get to your perfect body as quickly as possible.

Unfortunately, you aren't a simulation. Your goals need to be based in your reality. Trying to get everything perfect is a ticking time bomb for diet failure.

So, for flexible dieting to work, you need to find a balance between the results you want, how quickly you want them, and what you're willing and able to do to get them.

Saying you want to build 15 pounds of muscle and drop to 7% body fat as quickly as possible but you aren't willing to track your food or keep a strict diet is unrealistic.

Balancing your goals, reality, and the following three guidelines will lay the foundation for the amount of effort you need to apply to tracking and measuring—including what to track, when to track, when you don't need to track, and what will both make you happy and get you results.

As you read through everything in this section and apply everything in a later section, you will always need to weigh your desired results versus the flexibility you want in order to determine the accuracy and consistency you need to adhere to.

Guideline #2: Eat for Weight Change

What you eat will be the most significant determinant of your weight change. You can easily down a 1,000-calorie burger and fries in about 10 minutes, but burning 1,000 calories through exercise takes a lot of time and effort.

So, you need to eat the correct number of calories based on whether you want to boost muscle mass while minimizing fat gain or lower your body fat percentage while maintaining or increasing your muscle mass. This is your calorie surplus or deficit, better known as bulking or cutting, respectively.

In other words, eat the correct quantity of food to hit your recommended daily calories based on your weight-change goals.

You can also eat for weight change through nutrient partitioning by eating the correct nutrients to improve your health and help you store more body mass as muscle instead of fat.

Guideline #3: Eat to Build Muscle

Aside from eating the correct number of calories, it's better to focus on everything that helps you build muscle instead of everything that helps you lose fat.

This starts with eating enough high-quality protein every day to provide your body with the amino acids it needs to build muscle.

And this goes hand in hand with eating for weight change. Your body requires energy to build muscle, so taking in the correct number of calories will help you build muscle and train intensely.

Plus, building muscle is a very energy-intensive process, and your metabolic rate (calories burned daily while at rest) is heavily determined by the amount of lean body mass you have (more lean mass means more effortless fat loss).

So, when dieting, simply try to hit your daily calorie and protein requirements, and you'll get most of your results.

Guideline #4: Improve Diet Quality

Eating the correct number of calories and amount of protein will give you great results in the short term. But the longer a diet goes, the harder it will be to hit those guidelines if you're always hungry or eating only chicken, broccoli, and brown rice.

This fourth guideline means a majority of the food you eat should be "healthy." Try to get 75%–80% of your calories and macronutrients from plant-based whole foods and lean complete protein sources.

This is a transition from simply hitting calories and macros to improving your overall diet quality by eating foods that are better for you and are more conducive to a sustainable diet.

Diet quality and diet sustainability are two sides of the same coin. A diet's quality is determined by satiety, nutrient variety, and nutrient density.

Increasing the sustainability of a diet is done by gradually incorporating a variety of healthy and satiating foods into a structured, balanced, and flexible diet.

As you can probably tell, both require satiety. Satiety, or how full a diet makes you feel, can be the deciding factor in how long you will stick with a diet while also not hating life.

Satiety involves feeling full from the food you're eating so that even if you're eating less than usual, you aren't constantly feeling hungry and food-deprived.

Diet adherence largely depends on hunger, and hunger is a function of satiety.

You will simultaneously improve your results and your happiness by including more satiating foods rather than creating a restrictive diet, while you also prioritize building muscle and eating for weight change.

◇◇◇

As we take a look at the different nutrition variables and create a meal plan, keep these four guidelines for a flexible diet in mind. If you can hit each of them and follow the dieting hierarchy, you'll have a much more relaxed, enjoyable, and transformative diet.

CHAPTER 10

HOW MUCH TO EAT FOR THE PERFECT CUT OR BULK

As you know by now, weight change is heavily based on the calories you consume versus the calories you burn. In fact, energy balance is the most important factor to consider regarding your nutrition program.

Losing fat, building muscle, eating the correct foods for health, and timing your nutrients all draw from and rely on it. You can't correctly apply the other aspects of a nutrition program without first establishing your proper energy intake, i.e., the number of calories to eat.

This also means that when in dieting doubt, you should always revert back to determining how many calories you're eating and drinking and how many calories you're expending in a day, which you'll determine in this chapter.

As I mentioned in our discussion on the pillars of fat loss, scientists have come increasingly close to creating mathematical models that determine exactly how many calories a person burns daily. They can take specific information about a person and determine how many calories their body burns in a day based on their body, schedule, training, diet quality, gender, and more.

Armed with these equations and other research on adjusting your body fat and muscle mass, we can accurately determine how many calories you need to eat to change your weight however you like. You just need the correct equations, and you need to know how to use them. Unfortunately, many textbooks and other nutrition resources make this overly complicated or use completely inaccurate equations for determining how much to eat to achieve a quality cut or bulk.

I've blended simplicity and accuracy to give you the best formulas to use for optimal body recomposition without any unnecessary, overly scientific information, so you can concentrate on implementing them quickly and easily.

I know it sounds too good to be true, so let's look at the steps we'll take.

First, you need to determine your resting energy expenditure, or REE. Your REE is the number of calories you burn just by being alive, breathing, thinking, pumping blood, relaxing, etc., without training or doing anything else.

This is different and easier to determine than the commonly misrepresented basal metabolic rate (BMR).

Second, you'll figure out your total daily energy expenditure, or TDEE, by multiplying your resting energy expenditure by an activity adjustment factor (AF) based on how active you are throughout the day, including strength training.

Your TDEE is a very close approximation of the total number of calories you burn on an average day. This is also the number of calories you should eat on a maintenance diet to keep your weight the same.

Third, and finally, you'll multiply your TDEE by your optimal calorie deficit percentage to lose fat at the correct rate without sacrificing muscle and strength gains. Or, you'll multiply it by your optimal calorie surplus percentage to gain muscle without gaining too much body fat.

By figuring out your REE, translating it into your TDEE, and then figuring out how many calories you should eat to reach your weight-change goal, you can always easily and accurately estimate how many calories you should eat.

DETERMINE YOUR AVERAGE DAILY CALORIE EXPENDITURE

We will use a modified Ten Haaf formula to determine your resting energy expenditure because it is accurate, easy, and straightforward.

Twan ten Haaf and Peter Weijs determined their formula to be within 90%–95% accuracy for strength-training populations. Most other formulas that don't require knowing your body fat percentage or muscle mass (which are difficult to determine precisely) were only 40%–50% accurate.[1]

The original formula is overly complicated, so I rounded it slightly to make it easier to use to adjust your diet and calories each week.

Plus, your height and age won't change during a standard week. So, you can simply multiply your new weight in pounds by 5.45 (or in kilograms by 12) and add the rest of the equation that you already calculated.

Here is the slightly altered empirical formula:

$$\text{REE (calories)} = 5.45 \times \text{(weight in pounds)} + 15 \times \text{(height in inches)} - 8.16 \times \text{(age in years)} + 216$$

Here is the metric formula:

$$\text{REE (calories)} = 12 \times \text{(weight in kilograms)} + 590.4 \times \text{(height in meters)} - 8.16 \times \text{(age in years)} + 216$$

Next, we need to multiply your REE by an activity factor from the table below to determine how many calories you burn on an average day based on how active you are during the week.

This will give you your total daily energy expenditure, or the number of calories you burn in an average day. This is also your diet's maintenance calories.

The equation for turning your REE into your TDEE looks like this:

$$TDEE = REE \times AF$$

If you are training at the upper level of sets recommended in the training section and are lifting six days per week, you will most likely fall under "very active." Most people with less experience fall into the moderately active or lightly active category.

It's important to understand that the number of calories you burn while strength training is not dependent on how much weight you're lifting, how heavy you're breathing, or how fast you move from exercise to exercise.

When in doubt, use the lower activity factor number and adjust your calories based on the results you're getting. Here is the activity factor table:

Activity Level	Weekly Activity	Activity Factor (AF) Adjustment
Sedentary	Little or no exercise and a desk job	1.2
Lightly Active	Trains 1 to 3 days per week	1.35
Moderately Active	Trains 4 or 5 days per week	1.5
Very Active	Trains 6 or 7 days per week	1.7
Extremely Active	Very heavy exercise, a physical job, or training twice per day	1.85

THE THREE PHASES OF DIETING

In general, there are three phases of dieting: a cutting phase, a maintenance phase, and a lean bulking phase.

A proper "cut" is not a weight-loss diet; the goal is to lose fat while continuing to build muscle.

Similarly, "bulking" is not a "stuff-your-face" diet. Instead, when done correctly, it should pack on muscle mass while minimizing fat gain as much as possible.

You need a specific calorie deficit or surplus for a quality cut or bulk. Without a number to shoot for, you could lose muscle or gain too much fat, which would leave you worse off than when you started.

This brings us to the age-old question: to cut or to bulk?

I highly recommend that you spend most of your time rotating between the cutting and bulking phases. Then switch to a maintenance diet when you've reached your dream body or want to keep your body fat percentage very low for a short time, like during beach season.

Whether you should cut or "lean bulk" will depend on your current body fat percentage, along with your personal aesthetic preferences.

Research has shown that nutrient partitioning and overall health markers, which correlate to the ability to build muscle and lose fat, are optimal around 8%–12% body fat.

For reference and to help you approximate when to cut or bulk, at around 10%–15% body fat, most males will lose their lower-belly "pudge."

So, if you are above about 12% body fat, then you will cut first to optimize your body's ability to build muscle and improve standard health markers.

If you are at 12% body fat or slightly below, i.e., your lower-belly fat has disappeared, then you have a few options.

First, you can continue to cut until you reach a body fat percentage that gives you the body you want without sacrificing your health.

Your second option is to start a lean bulking phase. Energy intake has a minimal effect on muscle growth—but it still has an effect.

So, if you are already lean enough, it can be advantageous to lean bulk to ensure that you provide enough energy to your body for maximal muscle protein synthesis.

Finally, if you want to maintain your low body fat percentage but relax your diet and continue to build muscle, you can start a maintenance phase, or, if you feel inclined, you can call it "gaintenance" or "maingaining."

The next step is determining your optimal deficit or surplus for each phase.

The Cutting Phase

Calorie deficit (12% body fat or higher) = 10%-25% TDEE

Calorie deficit (7%-12% body fat) = 10% TDEE

The exact size of the calorie deficit that you should be in when attempting a cut will be based on how much body fat you have to lose. The higher your body fat percentage, the greater the deficit you can have without worrying about losing muscle mass.

Research has even shown that overweight individuals can be in a 50% calorie deficit from their total daily energy expenditure without excess muscle loss or adverse effects, since their body has a lot of stored calories to draw from—though you shouldn't do this without professional monitoring.

Similarly, the speed at which you lose body fat won't have much of an effect on your body, muscle building, metabolism, or energy levels, but it can greatly affect your hunger. So, you also need to consider whether a larger or smaller calorie deficit would be optimal for your hunger levels and diet adherence.

The lower your body fat percentage, the less of a calorie deficit you should be in. This lets you eat enough nutrients for a healthy diet while reducing the chance that taking in too few calories will hurt your metabolism or cause your muscles to break down.

That being said, we will implement two different cutting strategies.

The first strategy I simply call "the cut." The goal is to reduce your body fat percentage to approximately 12%. This phase is usually the longest, especially if you have a fairly high percentage of body fat, but it doesn't require as much accuracy.

If you are above 12% body fat, you will cut your calories by 10%–25% of your TDEE. The cut size will depend on your hunger levels, how rapidly you want results, and your diet adherence. However, the closer you get to 12% body fat, the lower your deficit should be, i.e., 20% maximum.

The goal at this stage of the cut is to form a simple and sustainable eating routine.

The second strategy is what I call "the shred," because you will cut your body fat to single digits. It requires much more accuracy to cut your body fat percentage from 12% to around 7%–8% without losing muscle or sacrificing your health and happiness.

When you get below 12% body fat, you should cut your calories by only 10% at most. You can perform a 10% cut until you get to 7%–8% body fat—where there is a clear separation between your muscles, and striations may start to appear.

The Lean Bulking Phase

Calorie surplus (7%-12% body fat) = 10% TDEE

The lean bulk is recommended for men with between 7% and 12% body fat who want to maximize their muscle-building efforts while also increasing their overall size and who don't mind adding a little bit of extra body fat in the process.

So, whether to bulk or go into a maintenance phase depends on your personal preferences. However, I recommend being in either a cut or a bulk, since it gives you a goal to strive for and you will always be looking to improve yourself.

If you choose to lean bulk, you will only slightly increase your total daily calories, by 10%. The goal here is to maximize muscle gain while minimizing fat gain.

Excessive calorie intake will only ramp up fat gain without increasing muscle gain.

While bulking, you will need to test your program and track your results for a week or two to determine whether you are gaining fat or muscle. Then adjust your program by another 10% if you're not getting the results you want.

How to Turn the Cut and Lean Bulk Phases Into Calories

Once you have your optimal cutting or bulking percentage, you need to turn this into the number of calories you should eat daily.

First, determine the percentage of calories you'll be consuming compared to your average energy expenditure. For example, if you are at about 20% body fat, you can implement a 25% calorie deficit. This means you are eating 75% of your maintenance calories (100% - 25% = 75%).

Next, multiply this percentage (75% in the example) by the number of calories you burn on an average day (your TDEE) to determine how many calories to eat each day. So, if your TDEE is 3,000 calories, you will eat 75% of that, or 2,250 calories a day.

Use these equations:

$$\text{Optimal weight-loss calorie intake} = \text{TDEE} \times (1 - \text{optimal deficit \%})$$

$$\text{Optimal weight-gain calorie intake} = \text{TDEE} \times (1 + \text{initial energy surplus \%})$$

At this point, you could be good to go for life by consistently switching between a cut and a lean bulk based on your preference, your goals, the different seasons, etc.

Or, you could use the third phase of dieting—the gaintenance or maingaining phase.

The Gaintenance/Maingaining Phase

If you are lean and don't want to gain any body fat for one reason or another, you will enter a maintenance phase. You will keep only your body fat percentage the same, not your weight, and hopefully not your muscle mass either.

The maintenance phase is perfect for enjoying the fruits of your labor. You can loosen up on your diet and figure out how many calories you need by using methods that work only for lean strength trainers.

However, you will need to work to maintain this state. You wouldn't want to work that hard to get to a low body fat percentage just to rebound back up. But this shouldn't worry you; maintenance is far easier than cutting.

Multiplying your body weight by a calorie-per-pound or calorie-per-kilogram factor is the easiest way to determine how many calories you need to eat for maintenance. Here is the table with the factors to use based on your training level:

Workouts per Week	3 or 4 (Beginner)	5 or More (Experienced)
Calories/lb	15	19
Calories/kg	33	42

So, if your weight has moved from 220 pounds to 150 pounds and you want to maintain it, you will take 150 pounds × 15 calories/pound = 2,250 calories.

Therefore, you will need to consume a total of 2,250 calories daily to maintain your weight.

This doesn't mean you'll remain at exactly 150 pounds for the rest of your life. Your weight may fluctuate, but the fluctuation will not be huge, and you can easily do a micro-cut or micro-bulk once you notice you are losing or gaining fat or muscle.

◇◇◇

Now that you know the number of calories you need to eat each day, you need to determine where those calories are coming from. The next chapter will convert the calories into protein, carbohydrates, and dietary fats.

CHAPTER 11

MACRONUTRIENTS FOR OPTIMAL MUSCLE GROWTH AND FAT LOSS

Knowing how many calories you should eat daily based on your weight-change goals is only one of the pillars of fat loss.

If you were to base a meal plan on energy balance alone (calories in versus calories out), you could get results, but the major change in your body would be in total mass—not necessarily fat loss and muscle gain.

For most, the goal isn't just to make the needle on the bathroom scale move up or down. The goal is to maximize your muscle-building potential while minimizing your total body fat percentage. This leaves you with a completely different body composition that is lean, muscular, and aesthetically pleasing.

In this chapter, we will add to the previous chapter by introducing the second and third pillars for weight change, along with the third pillar for building muscle.

In other words, we will take your recommended total daily energy intake and turn it into macronutrients. This is often called "hitting your macros."

These macronutrient recommendations are just that—recommendations. They will allow you to track your macronutrient intake and form a healthy diet. Yet trying to match every single macro exactly isn't necessary.

As you'll see, dietary fat intake is recommended to be 20%–40% of your total calories, carbohydrates don't have an exact recommendation, and protein has an optimal range of 1.6 to 1.8 grams per kilogram per day (g/kg/day).

So, you can "hit your macros" by having a diet that is 40% dietary fat and has 1.6 g/kg/day of protein with fruits and vegetables being used to hit the correct calorie recommendations, or you can have a diet that is higher in carbs and includes 20% dietary fat and 1.8 g/kg/day of protein.

There are no magic macronutrient profiles you need to hit. Instead, take each as a recommendation and allow for adjustments from day to day.

OPTIMAL PROTEIN INTAKE

Protein is responsible for building, repairing, and maintaining your body's tissues, including muscle. It is also the most satiating nutrient, which is very beneficial for weight loss and calorie restriction.

In order to build the most muscle mass possible, you will need to consume enough protein every day. If you fail to do this, your body won't have enough amino acids for muscle protein synthesis, i.e., muscle growth.

Eating excessive amounts of protein has no added benefits because the extra is just converted into energy or stored as body fat. And it can make eating enough healthy carbohydrates and fats difficult.

Determining the amount of protein you should eat in a day is filled with a lot of bro science and confusion.

The FDA recommends only 0.36 gram per pound of body weight per day (g/lb/d), or 0.8 g/kg/d, of protein for the average person to survive.

On one hand, the FDA's recommended intake for the average person is very low, because they need protein only in order to survive, not to build muscle.

On the other hand, the average bro-bodybuilder will have the view that training harder and consuming more protein will only result in more muscle.

While excessive protein consumption might be beneficial for professional bodybuilders on steroids, it isn't optimal for us natural strength trainees.

When it comes to muscle building and body recomposition, the upper limit of protein that your body can use is 0.73 g/lb/d, or 1.6 g/kg/d.

This is true whether you are male or female, train harder, are more or less advanced, have more or less muscle, are cutting or bulking, or any of the other reasons people say they need more protein.

To prove this, a meta-analysis, or a study of studies, of all the research available showed that there is no benefit to strength and muscle development by going above 1.6 g/kg/d; but, to be certain that you do get enough amino acids and to make up for the possibility of variation and the possibility of slight inaccuracy in the 49 different studies, a buffer is added to the upper-limit number.[1]

So, the recommended amount of protein you should consume per day is 0.82 gram per pound of your body weight, or 1.8 grams per kilogram of your body weight.[2] If you are a vegetarian or vegan, you may want to increase your intake by at least 10%.

Anything between 1.6 and 1.8 g/kg/d will provide great results. But since protein is satiating and you will be training using heavy weights, use the upper range to ensure that you get enough protein.

Grams of protein = body weight in pounds × 0.82 g/lb

Grams of protein = body weight in kilograms × 1.8 g/kg

Once you determine the amount of protein your body needs each day, you will want to find out how many calories this equates to. The calculation is very simple: 1 gram of protein is equivalent to 4 calories.

Calories from protein = grams protein × 4 calories per gram

OPTIMAL DIETARY FAT INTAKE

Among the three macronutrients, dietary fats are the densest sources of energy. Fat has 9 calories per gram, while carbs and proteins have only 4 calories per gram.

Ideally, dietary fats (from "good" fats) should make up 20%–40% of your total daily calories so that you can maximize your health and hormone development.

However, this recommendation is subjective, since there are no defined grounds on which dietary fat intake shows adverse effects. So, these percentage guidelines are not hard-and-fast rules. Instead, they should be seen as flexible and a place to start.

For that reason, I suggest that you try to get 30% of your daily calories from dietary fat, but you can easily bump this up to 40% if you want.

To calculate your daily dietary fat intake, simply multiply 30% (0.3) by your cutting or bulking daily calorie intake—which you calculated in the last chapter.

Calories from dietary fat = cutting/bulking calories × 0.3

Once you have your total daily calories from dietary fat, simply divide the calories by 9 to get the total grams of fat needed in a day.

Grams of daily fat = fat calories / 9 calories per gram

OPTIMAL CARBOHYDRATE INTAKE

Regardless of the source, almost all the food you eat is broken down to glucose and used or stored as energy to fuel your body. So, how many carbs you eat is less important than how much protein and fat you eat.

So, you only need to look to consume the correct amount of carbs for the health benefits that specific carbs provide (covered in the next chapter).

There are a few ways to determine your carbohydrate needs. But most of the time, it's best to set carbohydrate targets based on how many calories are left over after protein and fat targets have been set. The formula is as follows:

Carbohydrate target calories = total daily calories – protein calories – fat calories

---

Target grams of carbohydrates = carbohydrate target calories / 4 calories per gram

---

This makes it easier to adjust your carb intake based on your training goals. For instance, if you are on an eating plan and are getting the correct amounts of calories from fats and proteins, but you're not seeing the results you want, you can simply slowly add or subtract carbs until you start getting results.

WATER AND HYDRATION

Knowing that water is vital for survival, as well as for the structure and building of muscles, and that even mild dehydration can lead to poor exercise performance, it's often recommended that you drink a lot of water before, during, and after your workouts.

However, strength-training performance is generally not affected by mild to moderate dehydration. Many studies done on strength training and dehydration show that dehydration will only consistently impair exercise bouts and the ability to produce maximal force lasting longer than 30 seconds, which is longer than most strength-training sets take.[3]

In fact, to keep us from dying and to help keep our bodies working optimally, humans have developed an amazing mechanism to help us know when we need to gulp down a glass of water: thirst.[4]

Research has shown that simply drinking water in response to your natural thirst is the best way to prevent both dehydration and the adverse effects of overhydration.[5]

For strength-training sessions that last less than 90 minutes, all you need to do to stay hydrated is drink when you're thirsty.[6,7]

So, if you are not working out super-intensely, you're not a competitive athlete, and you aren't actively trying to dehydrate yourself, you can usually get away with drinking water when you are thirsty. You don't need to be excessive, but you do need to drink water.

I would suggest consuming at least a glass of water with every meal, but closer to 16 to 24 ounces (0.5 to 0.7 liter) at each meal. This will ensure that you drink enough water throughout the day, will make you feel fuller, and will keep you from consuming extra calories that you might otherwise take in in the form of another beverage, such as soda or alcohol.

◇◇◇

Many diets have been based on simply "hitting your macros." While the premise of "if it fits your macros," or IIFYM, can help you structure your diet and be cognizant of what you're eating, the assumption is that you have a perfect macronutrient profile determined.

Instead, as I mentioned at the beginning of the chapter, take each of these macronutrient targets—except for protein—as a recommendation. By hitting your daily protein requirements and your daily calories, and including healthy foods in your diet, you'll ensure that your macros will take care of themselves. This is the focus of the next chapter.

CHAPTER 12

WHAT TO EAT FOR OPTIMAL HEALTH AND SATIETY

It is true that your health is more important than anything else, but you need to understand that you don't need a perfect diet to be healthy.

Being healthy is more of a construct than a precise thing. Often, it's as much psychological as it is physiological, with the main health markers being determined by how you feel combined with what a blood test shows.

Consequently, there are thousands of different ways to become "healthy." Chasing a perfect diet that hits every single vitamin and mineral requirement, has the correct probiotics and prebiotics, and provides antioxidant, anti-inflammatory, and phytonutrients is a recipe for disaster (if not impossible).

So, to counteract this and help you learn enough to actually implement it, I'm going to keep this topic broad. We will only talk about food groups, which are made up of the macronutrient recommendations from the last chapter.

Remember, this is the third level of importance when it comes to implementation. Only once you can actually make a meal plan and add in healthy foods, versus cutting out unhealthy foods, should you even think about highly specific foods.

Above all, it's important to remember that strength training, building muscle, and being lean provide so many benefits that can outweigh the negative side effects of a mediocre diet.

So, by being "good enough" with your food sources, you'll be able to build an amazing body while being incredibly healthy—and do it with less stress and effort.

If you want to change your eating habits and start eating better foods, instead of cutting out and avoiding certain foods, try to add a variety of healthy and filling foods to your diet on a regular basis using the sources below.

IMPORTANT PROTEINS

The majority of your protein needs should be met by high-quality protein sources, followed by a variety of other protein sources. Protein quality is, more or less, determined by a food's ability to provide your body with the correct amino acid profile for muscle protein synthesis and not just energy creation.

High-quality protein sources are "complete proteins," which means they have the right amounts of all the amino acids for health and growth and can be absorbed and used for growth.

Proteins in your diet can be from both plants and animals, but the proteins from animals are generally considered to be of higher quality. Animal proteins contain an excellent amino acid profile for humans to build muscles and have better digestibility and bioavailability than plant-based food sources.

You should try to consume a variety of animal and plant protein sources to take advantage of each source's different nutrients. Also, by getting enough protein from mixed sources (animal and plant), you'll have a less monotonous diet while ensuring that you hit all of your body's essential amino acid requirements.

Animal-Based Proteins

Try to get most of your total daily protein from unprocessed, lean, animal-based protein food sources (unless you are vegan or vegetarian), such as poultry, pork, low-fat dairy products, and lean fish.

To round out your micronutrient intake, you should also include, though less often, whole milk and dairy products, whole eggs, red meat, and fatty fish and shellfish—especially oily and fatty fish and shellfish. If possible, eat fatty fish like salmon, mackerel, and sardines three to five times every week for an adequate supply of omega-3 essential fatty acids.

Red meat is a very good source of iron, zinc, and other nutrients needed for proper body function—all of which are better absorbed by our bodies than iron and zinc from plant foods.

Egg yolks are our primary source of choline, a B vitamin that is critically important for the health of brain cells.

Dairy-based foods contain calcium and vitamin D, which are vital for bone formation, muscle contraction, and improved mental health.

As long as you eat a variety of animal-based protein sources, you shouldn't worry too much about which sources you add to your diet.

Plant-Based Proteins

Multiple plant-based foods contain decent amounts of protein. These foods include beans or legumes, nuts, seeds, soy, and grains.

However, soy is the only plant-based protein source considered a complete protein. Therefore, you need to ensure that you are eating enough animal protein or consuming complementary plant-based protein sources.

Complementary proteins are two or more protein-rich foods that combine to form a complete protein source.

To ensure that you meet your body's amino acid requirements, mix and match your protein sources so that foods low in one essential amino acid are balanced by foods high in the same amino acid.

In general, a diet containing 50% protein from legumes (pea protein, soy products, beans, and lentils), 25% protein from seeds (hemp, chia, and sunflower seeds), and 25% protein from grains (rice and wheat protein) will provide a good amino acid profile.

But keep in mind that plant-based proteins are also less digestible and bioavailable, so vegans and vegetarians need to increase their daily protein requirements by at least 10%, most likely more.

Consuming enough protein as a vegan or vegetarian can be very difficult, so it's recommended that you include an 80-20 pea-to-rice protein powder mix.

If you choose to go meatless, make sure to carefully plan your diet to avoid nutritional deficiencies. Meatless diets frequently have low levels of calcium, creatine, iron, zinc, vitamin B, vitamin D, and the omega-3 fatty acids DHA and EPA.

IMPORTANT CARBOHYDRATES

Since your body can make glucose from proteins and fats, carbohydrate requirements for a quality diet are based on consuming enough nutrients for your health.

Aim for 75%–80% of your carbohydrate intake to be from unprocessed, whole foods, with a focus on a variety of fruits and vegetables first, followed by other fibrous foods, and starchy carbs last. These foods are very filling, have a good ratio of nutrients to calories, and are full of vitamins, minerals, phytochemicals, and fiber that your body needs.

With 75%–80% of your foods as close to their natural state as possible, you can fill your diet with nutrient-dense and satiating foods while still being able to include "less-healthy" processed foods.

Fruits and Vegetables

You should fill your meal plan with fruits and vegetables before any other carb source.

Different people have different ideas about how much of each you should eat every day, depending on things like your own needs and the type of fruit or vegetable.

A basic rule of thumb is to try to eat both a serving of fruits and a serving of vegetables for about every 500 to 750 calories in your diet. So, if you have a 2,000-calorie diet, you should eat about three to four servings of each daily.

This can be done by eating a serving or two of both fruits and vegetables at every meal or eating multiple servings of fruits in one meal and multiple servings of vegetables in another. For example, an orange by itself and blueberries on oatmeal for breakfast, an apple by itself and spinach on a sandwich for lunch, and multiple servings of asparagus for dinner.

In general, try to eat a lot of different fruits and vegetables every day. This will give your body a wide range of micronutrients and help you avoid nutrient deficiencies.

Fiber-Rich Foods

Research has shown that men should consume at least 35 grams of dietary fiber daily to reap all of the health benefits it provides.[1]

Foods like whole grains, brown rice, oats, fruits, vegetables, and legumes (beans) are great sources of fiber.

Prioritizing eating enough fiber is huge for fat loss and overall health. Fiber provides great satiation, which helps prevent hunger and possible overeating, and it increases the amount of calories you burn in a day through digestion.

In addition, high-fiber diets have been shown to improve digestion, the immune system, and glucose control, and they lower blood pressure and cholesterol to reduce the risk of cardiovascular diseases. In fact, high fiber intake has been shown to decrease mortality rates by up to 30%.[2]

You don't need to worry about whether the fiber you're getting is soluble or insoluble; that just adds more work for very little reward.

Starches

Starch is the storage form of glucose in plants. Starch is to plants what glycogen is to humans. These are your classic "complex carbs."

The most common starches are corn, seeds, grains, rice, peas, beans, and potatoes.

Starches often get a bad rap as not being very nutritious, but this is not completely accurate. Some starches are very high in nutrients, and most people can use starches to make meals that are both tasty and healthy.

Once you've put your fruits, vegetables, and other high-fiber foods into your plan, you should add starches to meet the rest of your unprocessed carbohydrate needs.

IMPORTANT DIETARY FATS

In general, if the majority of your food choices are plant-based from a variety of vegetables, fruits, whole grains, beans, nuts, and seeds, and you add in lean-animal-protein-rich food sources (fish, meat, and dairy), your total fat intake will most likely be in a well-controlled zone of about 20%–40% of your daily calories.

This lets you focus on getting more healthy fats into your diet without having to worry about any negative effects. If your calorie intake is correct, you'll only get more benefits.

If you want to eat fats that will help you maximize your results and feel your best, look for unsaturated fats from oils, olives, nuts, and avocados and increase your intake of omega-3 fatty acids.

Unsaturated Fatty Acids

Try to make unsaturated fat your primary fat source. Unsaturated fats are liquid at room temperature, most often in the form of oils.

Polyunsaturated fats are liquids at room temperature, and they remain liquids even when subjected to low temperatures. Polyunsaturated fats are abundant in foods like sesame, corn, sunflower seeds, and many nuts.

Monounsaturated fats are liquids at room temperature, but they can become solids when subjected to low temperatures. Foods that are high in monounsaturated fats include olives, avocados, and peanut oil.

You should look to consume both monounsaturated and polyunsaturated fats, but you don't need to be concerned about the ratio between the two.

Essential Fatty Acids

Essential fatty acids are a type of polyunsaturated fatty acid that our bodies can't make on their own. This means we have to get them from food or supplements in order to stay healthy and even prevent early death.

The two primary essential fatty acids are:

- Alpha-linolenic acid (ALA)

- Linoleic acid (LA)

ALA is found primarily in leafy vegetables, and LA is found primarily in corn and peanut oils.

From LA, your body can produce the omega-6 fatty acids known as gamma-linolenic acid and arachidonic acid (no need to memorize).

Similarly, your body can make the omega-3 fatty acids eicosapentaenoic acid (EPA) and docosa-hexaenoic acid (DHA) from ALA.

The omega-3 fatty acids ALA, EPA, and DHA are the most important when it comes to losing fat and building muscle.

An abundance of research on omega-3s and omega-6s shows that a diet with a higher ratio of omega-3 fatty acids to omega-6s has tremendous health benefits for your body.[3] This could be the reason some people consider the effects of omega-6s to be generally "bad" and those of omega-3s as generally "good."

However, research conducted on the inflammatory effects of both fatty acids showed that, while omega-3s are anti-inflammatory, omega-6s are not pro-inflammatory, contrary to common belief.[4] In fact, that same study showed that omega-6 fatty acids can decrease your risk of heart disease.

That's why scientists recommend just consuming enough omega-3s rather than being too concerned about the ratio of omega-3s to omega-6s.

Omega-3 Fatty Acids

Omega-3 fatty acids have been shown to improve cognition, reduce depression, provide joint protection, decrease fat mass, increase lean body mass and muscle growth, and more.[5,6] Clearly, given the long list of benefits of omega-3s, they are important to include in your diet.

For maximal benefits, you should look to consume at least 500 milligrams of EPA and DHA from food (fatty fish) daily or 750 milligrams from high-quality supplements. However, you will benefit more from an omega-3 intake of around 2 grams per day from approximately 700 grams of fatty fish per week, or 3 grams of EPA and DHA fish oil supplements per day.

If you eat fish three to five times a week, as suggested in the discussion of protein sources above, you should get the recommended amount of omega-3 fatty acids. If you don't get this much fish, you might need to take a supplement.

Saturated Fatty Acids

Saturated fats have long been misunderstood, leading to their being associated with clogged arteries, heart attacks, diabetes, and more. Actually, many studies and meta-analyses have found no correlation between saturated fats and coronary heart disease, stroke, blood cholesterol levels, fat gain, or type 2 diabetes.[7,8]

In reality, saturated fatty acids help your body make anabolic hormones and cholesterol, both of which have positive effects on muscle growth.

Cholesterol follows very closely behind saturated fats when it comes to being misunderstood. Yet it is cholesterol that is the biggest help with anabolic hormone production, because cholesterol is the precursor of anabolic hormones.

However, you should still limit your saturated fat intake to only about 10% of your total daily calorie intake—though don't go out of your way to completely avoid this fat, as it is still beneficial for your health and strength-training goals.

Saturated fats are mostly solid at room temperature—think butter and solid fats.

This includes fatty meats, egg yolks, whole dairy products, and more—plus most processed and premade meals or foods.

You shouldn't have to worry about affecting your blood cholesterol levels if you limit your saturated fat intake to 10% of your daily calorie intake, though research has shown that there is no correlation between blood cholesterol levels and saturated fat intake.[9,10,11]

All in all, if you don't have diabetes or a cardiovascular disease, your diet is healthy without overly processed meats or foods, and you strength train, the amount of cholesterol in your diet is unlikely to be a concern.[12]

To be safe, you should get your cholesterol levels checked every few years, even if you have no known reason for concern.

◇◇◇

As you can see, creating a "healthy" diet doesn't need to be overly difficult. The standard foods that your mom and elementary school teachers have repeatedly told you to eat more of will end up making up most of a quality diet.

The real key will be to ensure that you have a variety of these different food sources; you include satiating foods to keep you full during the day; and you focus on foods that are good for you without feeling the need to exclude other foods.

In an upcoming section, we'll go over different types of foods based on the broad categories we discussed in this chapter. Then we'll place them into an actual meal plan so you can see how everything comes together.

CHAPTER 13

THE TRUTH ABOUT NUTRIENT TIMING FOR ACCELERATING YOUR RESULTS

Pre-workout and post-workout nutrition programming has become overhyped over the years. Supplement companies have paid millions of dollars to get you to believe that if you don't chug down a whey protein shake with maltodextrin within 30 minutes of a workout, your whole session was a waste of time. You will have completely missed the "anabolic window" directly after your workout, when your muscles are being broken down by cortisol from your training and are highly receptive to protein.

To get your body to switch from breaking down muscle to building muscle, they say, you clearly need fast-acting carbs and fast-digesting protein. So, if you don't buy their whey protein and sugar for the price of steak, your time in the gym will be worthless.

For the sake of your wallet and physique, you need to understand that you've been lied to—the anabolic window for most people lasts 24 hours or more, protein makes carbs redundant, and your body has a lot of stored energy to get you through your workout.

Instead, here is what you need to know and be aware of.

PRE-WORKOUT PROTEIN

The goal for most lifters is to provide a steady supply of amino acids over the whole day.

To help with this, you should consume 30 to 40 grams of protein within 2 hours before your workout. This keeps your muscles from breaking down and gives them a steady supply of amino acids for protein synthesis, which leads to more muscle growth.

There is no need to overcomplicate pre-workout protein timing. Simply eat a high-protein meal relatively close to your workout time and you'll be good to go.

POST-WORKOUT PROTEIN AND THE "ANABOLIC WINDOW"

Your muscles are much more sensitive to amino acids after a training session. They are like dry sponges that are ready to soak up more amino acids than normal.

This heightened responsiveness to protein is termed the "anabolic window." In spite of what most people think, your body doesn't increase muscle protein synthesis during the anabolic window.

Instead, it is a period of delayed muscle fullness that can result in more protein synthesis over time. By being able to take in more amino acids than usual and being more sensitive to them, you can create more potential for muscle growth.

So, it's important to consume protein post-workout, within your anabolic window, to increase the potential for muscle growth.

While supplement companies tell you to chug down their whey protein powder within 30 to 60 minutes after your workout to avoid missing your anabolic window, research has shown that the anabolic window is actually about 10 hours for advanced lifters and all the way to 72 hours for novice lifters.

So, for optimal results, you should eat 30 to 40 or more grams of protein within 1 to 2 hours after your workout is finished. However, there is no need to rush to do this, because your pre-workout protein will still be digesting and reaching your muscle cells for about 6 hours.

If you eat protein 2 hours pre-workout, then spend 2 hours working out plus traveling to and from the gym and warming up, and then eat within 2 hours post-workout, you will be within this 6-hour window and ensure that you consume enough protein to work with your anabolic window.

PRE-WORKOUT CARBS (MINIMAL NEEDED)

Since you will be consuming protein pre-workout and your muscles store glucose for usable energy to prevent excess muscle breakdown, you do not need more than 10 to 20 grams of carbs (source is unimportant) before a workout to ensure that you can train optimally while also supporting maximum muscle growth.[1]

The idea behind eating carbs before a workout is to make sure your body has energy to burn right away and that your glycogen stores don't become depleted, which would lead to a mediocre workout.

Except your body is very good at regulating glycogen levels, because running out of muscle glycogen would be detrimental to your system.[2] If you train intensely, your body synthesizes glycogen faster. And if you seriously deplete your glycogen stores, your body will store more glycogen for the future.

As an example, a study was done in which participants performed sets of leg extensions until they reached absolute failure (yet they still couldn't completely deplete their glycogen stores). Afterward, the participants were not allowed to consume anything. Yet, within 6 hours, their bodies had already restored 75% of their muscles' glycogen.[3]

So, research has shown that for best results, you need only 10 to 20 grams of carbs before strength training.

POST-WORKOUT CARBS (NOT NEEDED)

The premise behind consuming post-workout simple carbs is to create an insulin spike that halts muscle protein breakdown and shuttles amino acids directly into your muscles.

To put it simply, insulin "unlocks" a cell's wall, allowing glucose, amino acids, and other nutrients to flood into the cell. This initiates the anabolic process of repair, which suppresses the catabolic process of muscle protein breakdown.

Carbs can't stimulate muscle protein synthesis because, well, they're not proteins. But, by stimulating insulin production, which is called being insulinogenic, they can have an anticatabolic effect.

Less breakdown and more nutrients would theoretically mean more muscle growth, right?

Except theories don't always pan out. First, your body doesn't like to break down muscle protein, so this process doesn't occur as much as is touted in supplement advertisements.

Second, carbohydrates aren't the only macronutrient that initiates the release of insulin. High-quality protein sources are also highly insulinogenic, and it takes only about 20 grams of protein to break the insulin threshold for maximum suppression of muscle protein breakdown.[4]

Basically, what this means is that by eating enough protein, you make post-workout carb consumption redundant.

One group of researchers wanted to test this exact argument. The study concluded: "Whole body protein breakdown, synthesis, and oxidation rates, as well as whole body protein balance, did not differ between experiments. . . . In conclusion, co-ingestion of carbohydrates during recovery does not further stimulate post-exercise muscle protein synthesis when ample protein is ingested."[5]

Many other studies have been conducted following this, and they all came to the same conclusion: chugging simple carbohydrates post-workout only adds more calories to your diet.

TIMING DIETARY FATS (NOT NEEDED)

Dietary fats don't need to be consumed at any specific time to help maximize muscle-growth or fat-loss potential, or provide energy for hard training. Simply consume an adequate amount of dietary fat throughout the day.

Fats have little to no effect on the absorption rate of protein, muscle protein breakdown prevention, protein synthesis rates upon consumption, or rapid energy production.

◇◇◇

As you can see, nutrient timing is grossly overhyped for strength trainers, thanks largely to supplement companies.

Simply consume protein and at least a little bit of carbs pre-workout to prevent possible muscle breakdown.

Then eat protein within about 2 hours post-workout and you'll be good to go.

Stressing about eating fast-acting whey protein as soon as you finish a workout isn't necessary, and post-workout protein makes post-workout carbs redundant.

CHAPTER 14

HOW TO SCHEDULE YOUR MEALS AND NUTRIENTS TO PUT YOUR LIFE ON AUTOPILOT

Life is hectic. We are all busy, get distracted, and have to keep track of multiple things at once, and it often feels like there is never enough time in a day to accomplish all that we need to do. With very long to-do lists that, in all likelihood, we'll take with us to the grave, sticking to determined calories and macronutrients can feel impossible—but it doesn't have to.

To succeed in your muscle-building and fat-loss goals, you just need to form a sustainable routine that lets your day consistently run smoothly. Having a routine and a structured eating schedule helps reduce decision fatigue, reduces meal-prep stress, and allows you to prepare your meals ahead of time—so you can spend more time doing the things you enjoy while being mentally present for them.

But you shouldn't change your eating schedule until you can figure out your calorie intake accurately and consistently, get at least your daily protein intake, and include healthier and more satiating foods in your diet.

Eating a specific amount of protein within your "anabolic window" is worthless if everything else in your diet is out of whack.

Your diet routine should easily fit into your daily schedule, reduce your hunger levels, and make your life easier. It should also work with your strength training so you can get the right nutrients at the right times to help your muscles grow as much as possible.

Many people overcomplicate meal scheduling and nutrient timing, but if you follow the simple guidelines in this chapter, you will see that creating an eating schedule that revolves around you while still getting you amazing results is far easier and more enjoyable than most people think.

SUSTAINABLE MEAL STRUCTURE CONSIDERATIONS

Consume Three or Four Large Meals per Day

Eating raises your metabolism because your body uses energy to digest your food. We've talked about this thermic effect of food (TEF)—the total increase in your metabolism and total calories burned during digestion.

If you eat healthy, complete meals, this effect can increase the number of calories you burn in a day by a couple of hundred.

Eating many smaller meals during the day creates frequent small spikes in your metabolism, like adding kindling to a campfire.

On the other hand, eating fewer, larger meals is like placing a log on the fire. It creates larger and longer spikes due to the increased digestion time.

When calories and protein are equal, eating many small meals burns the same number of calories during digestion and results in the same fat loss and the same muscle growth as simply eating normal meals three or four times a day.

However, eating only three or four meals a day has been shown to help with diet adherence and ensure that you eat enough food during meals to fill you up. It's also easy to plug into most people's schedules. Few people have the time to prepare and eat five or six meals a day, every day.

So, in scheduling your diet, simply plan for three or four larger meals a day at your regular eating times.

Eat Mixed Meals

Mixed meals are meals that contain all three of the macronutrients. When you eat a mixed meal that includes unprocessed sources of protein, carbohydrates, and dietary fat, your body has to work harder to digest all the macronutrients at the same time.

It's like trying to sort Legos as you take apart something you've built. If all the Legos are the same color, you just need to pull them apart. But if there are multiple colors of Legos, sorting becomes a bit more difficult.

Digesting mixed meals burns more calories and increases the TEF—much more so than just eating each macronutrient by itself. Plus, mixed meals are much more satiating than protein, fat, or carbs separately.

In other words, mixed meals made of whole foods keep you fuller longer and burn more calories during digestion. That's a win-win for fat loss and diet sustainability.

So, chugging down that protein shake might keep calories low and increase the amount of protein you're getting in your diet, but it will burn far fewer calories during digestion and will be less filling than just eating an actual meal.

Eat Similar Meals Each Day

To cut down on the time and stress of deciding what to eat and the amount of time it takes to prepare different things for every single meal every day, you should eat similar meals each day.

Often, stress overeating (which is completely normal) can be prevented, or at least minimized, by being organized and knowing in advance what you're going to eat. This means having already-prepared meals, knowing what you're going to eat or prepare next, and sticking to your eating schedule.[1]

Also, by sticking to a similar meal structure but slightly adjusting the types of foods, you will have an easy-to-follow meal plan with enough variety for long-term adherence. For example, if you eat a turkey sandwich and an apple every day, you can easily swap the turkey for chicken and the apple for a handful of berries.

This also allows for easy weekly meal preparation and planning meals ahead of time, allowing you to have more time to focus on other important things in your life—like family, friends, work, etc.

Adjust Your Eating Times to Match Your Hunger

You need to stick to regular eating times, but it can be beneficial to adjust when you eat your meals and the different sizes of your meals based on your natural hunger.

By moving your meal times around based on when you get hungry without worrying about having to eat at certain times because it is the societal norm, you can reduce hunger and snacking and make dieting easier.

You can also take it a step further by adjusting your meal sizes to match your hunger. Allocate more food to meals when you're naturally hungriest (or post-workout) and make your other meals slightly smaller.

For example, if you wake up in the morning and normally eat breakfast at 8:00 a.m. before starting work, even though you normally aren't hungry until 11:00 a.m., then you could bump back your first meal to 11:00 a.m., sidestep snacking in the afternoon by eating your lunch at 3:00 p.m., and eat your dinner at 8:00 p.m. to avoid snacking before bed.

Plus, if you normally overeat during dinner, you can backload your calories and make that final meal of the day much larger.

A person who doesn't get hungry at night but is ravenous in the morning would have the opposite schedule.

All in all, as long as you eat at the same times each day, the exact hours when you have your meals aren't overly important.

HOW TO SCHEDULE YOUR MEALS

Now that you know your optimal daily calorie intake for cutting or bulking, and you've turned the calories into your daily requirements for protein, carbs, and fats, you need to place everything into a schedule that works for you.

As we discussed, you need a sustainable diet that you can form a routine around. Eating three or four larger mixed meals a day will result in the exact same fat loss and muscle gain as eating many smaller meals, but the former strategy is far easier to build a sustainable routine around.

Also, you need to sandwich your workout with about 30 to 40 grams of protein within 2 hours pre-workout and another 30 to 40 grams of protein within 2 hours post-workout. Therefore, you'll plan two of your three or four meals to bookend your normal workout time and will have a diet that fits your daily schedule.

To make your life easier for now, just split your macronutrients evenly among your meals. Then eat when you are normally hungry or have free time in your day.

For example, if you work out in the mornings, you can have a meal before working out (or even just a protein shake if you work out very early) and then eat at your normal lunch time. This would give you the 2-hour buffer you need.

If you wanted to follow a three-meal schedule, it could look like this:

> **Protein per meal = daily protein intake / 3 meals**
> **Carbs per meal = daily carb intake / 3 meals**
> **Fats per meal = daily fat intake / 3 meals**

> **7:00 a.m.: Meal 1**
> **9:00–10:00 a.m.: Workout**
> **12:00 p.m.: Meal 2**
> **6:00 p.m.: Meal 3**

Most people have a strict schedule due to work, so they eat breakfast before work, eat lunch on their lunch break, have a snack midafternoon, work out after work ends, and then eat dinner. In this case, splitting your macronutrients into four meals would be beneficial.

For example, if you work out after work, your eating schedule could be four meals split evenly and could be scheduled like this:

Protein per meal = daily protein intake / 4 meals
Carbs per meal = daily carb intake / 4 meals
Fats per meal = daily fat intake / 4 meals

8:00 a.m.: Meal 1
12:00 p.m.: Meal 2
4:00 p.m.: Meal 3
6:00–7:00 p.m.: Workout
8:00 p.m.: Meal 4

◇◇◇

Creating a schedule takes your ideal intakes and places them in a legitimate plan. A failure to plan is a plan to fail, and a goal without a plan is just a dream.

Your meal schedule should allow you to put your nutrition program on autopilot. You shouldn't have to be constantly concerned about what you're going to eat and when. It should be a second thought that only pops into your mind during meal prep or when a change in plans is needed due to unforeseen circumstances.

You will be able to cruise to better results with far less effort if you eat the same or similar foods every day; stick to strict eating times; eat large, satiating meals three or four times a day; consume 30 to 40 grams of protein 2 hours pre- and post-workout; and keep the rest of your daily schedule in check.

SECRET 5

-

HOW TO TRAIN TO TRANSFORM YOUR PHYSIQUE QUICKLY

CHAPTER 15

TURNING SIMPLE SCIENCE INTO OPTIMIZED TRAINING VARIABLES

By now, you should know that strength training is the key to building that fantastic physique you're after. All you need are the correct variables to plug into your program and the correct exercises to get you there (and some hard work, of course).

There are five things that a strength-training program needs in order to be effective. Each of these five things has specific training variables that correspond to it, which we will discuss throughout this section.

The goal of your strength-training program is to (1) provide an intense enough force and (2) enough volume (3) as frequently as possible (4) to consistently overload (5) a specific muscle so that all of its muscle fibers increase their size and ability to handle that force.

As you might have been able to tell, those are three of the pillars of building muscle: maximizing mechanical tension, progressively overloading your muscles, and providing enough recovery time.

Many things directly affect how much tension your muscles receive and how well you can progressively overload your body, even outside of a single workout or a strength-training program. But learning every little detail about each variable and how to manipulate them all is not worth your time and effort. In reality, each part of a training program has an optimal range that will provide the best results for the vast majority of people.

This is where we will focus in this book. You're not reading this book to pass a test; you're reading this book to learn the best way to train and eat to build more muscle and strength and to get lean.

This means that each strength-training program variable can be highly specific to those exact results.

Throughout this section, I will outline the different variables that make up a strength-training program and discuss what research has shown are the best ways to apply them.

Anything outside the recommendations either doesn't work for building muscle and strength efficiently or has such a minimal effect that its costs outweigh its benefits.

THE ONE THING ALWAYS TO CONCENTRATE ON

Apart from following the programs of bro-scientists, fitness "influencers," bodybuilding magazines, etc., a lot of men struggle to get results because they treat training for strength differently than training for hypertrophy. Often, they will treat each training variable like it's not intertwined with anything else and base their training session on feeling, essentially switching from training to simply exercising with weights.

Creating a program by feel is like throwing darts at a dartboard while blindfolded in the hope that your guesstimated training variables are perfect for you.

I'm going to let you in on a little secret: designing an amazing strength-training program to create an amazing body is a delicate balancing act that takes years to learn.

Imagine a large balancing scale with a bunch of different measuring arms to place objects on. If you place more on one measuring arm than the others, the scale will become unbalanced and tip.

But if you place the same exact amount on each measuring arm, the scale will remain balanced, and you'll be able to place more and more on the scale. But again, even one little mismeasure would tip the scales and throw everything off.

This is the same idea we will follow when creating a strength-training program. There are a lot of variables that rely on each other, and if you don't keep everything balanced, the scale will eventually tip.

If you go too hard one day, your future workouts will suffer because you'll be too tired and sore, if not injured. Move from one exercise to the next as quickly as you can, and you'll be too worried about catching your breath to concentrate on lifting the most weight possible.

To keep your scale balanced while also growing and improving, thus building a better and better body, your goal should always be to try to increase your strength in some way. You will adjust every training program variable to increase your strength.

It doesn't matter if you don't care about getting strong and only care about being lean, healthy, or muscular; building a big chest; having a sculpted six-pack; or looking completely shredded. By getting stronger in one way or another, you will get the results you want.

CHAPTER 16

THE THREE MOST IMPORTANT TRAINING VARIABLES

The different variables that make up a training program are nothing more than a way to organize your workout so you can consistently improve your body.

Each variable plays a part in the amount and type of stress you place on your body, your body's ability and time to recover fully, and the type and speed of adaptations you get in return.

To optimize your muscle building and strength, the most important things to consider are the intensity of stress, volume of stress, and frequency with which stress is applied. In exercise science, these are referred to as your training intensity, volume, and frequency.

In fact, the muscle growth and strength improvement process will follow three major steps, which are all interconnected and reliant on each other.

First, you need to provide a large enough amount of stress so that each of a muscle's fibers receives tension. This is determined by your training intensity.

Training intensity will directly affect the amount of weight you use, the number of repetitions you can do of a specific exercise, the amount of tension your muscles receive at a given time, and your strength improvements. This is different from training intensiveness, or how taxing a workout is ("That was an intense workout").

Then you need to repeat this until your muscles and their fibers are stressed enough to want and need to improve neurologically, morphologically, and metabolically—which is determined by your training volume.

The goal is to train each muscle with enough volume to trigger muscle growth in each muscle fiber while avoiding overtraining and injuries from excessive volume. This is done by repeatedly performing an exercise with enough weight and reps (training intensity), i.e., doing enough sets per muscle per training session and week.

Finally, you need to bridge the gap between the amount of total stress you provide at one time and the amount of time you allow your muscles to recover before you repeat this process. Your training frequency per muscle will bridge this gap.

Simply put, training frequency is a measure of how many days per week you train a specific muscle.

You want to train each muscle often enough to increase the intensity per exercise, i.e., lift as much weight as possible and complete as many reps as possible. However, you also want to train with a frequency that allows you to do enough sets in a training session to trigger muscle growth.

In this chapter, we'll nail down your training volume, intensity, and frequency by establishing the perfect number of sets, the number of reps you complete per set, and how frequently to train each muscle so that you can consistently increase your strength and muscle mass.

These three training variables form the foundation for creating a training program. Therefore, they are the three most important variables to dial in and implement.

You can have the correct sets, reps, and frequency of a few core exercises and get great results by simply adjusting weight as needed, doing a variety of exercises that stress the correct muscle groups, resting as needed, and doing random routines for warming up and cardio.

There are a lot of men with incredible bodies who only strength train with the correct intensity, volume, and training frequency. Still, they get great results because they have these variables optimized.

Let's discuss each variable so you can place them into your strength-training program.

DO 12 TO 16 SETS PER MUSCLE

To build the most muscles possible, you will do 12 to 16 sets per muscle per week. This will give your body the perfect amount of stimulus for muscle growth without overtraining, undertraining, or needing to resort to guessing and checking.

It is very common for new and even experienced weight lifters to take a guess as to the number of sets to do, try that program for a few training sessions, and then adjust the number of sets randomly— either by adding more if they haven't noticed any results, or by removing some because their bodies ache and they're tired.

In the end, some people do far too many sets for their bodies to recover from, leading to injuries, overtraining, or just poor muscle growth. Others don't do enough sets to trigger growth in their targeted muscles and will never see the gains they want.

For optimal strength and muscle development, you should stick with the research- and real-world-backed range of 12 to 16 sets per week for each muscle.

To reach these totals per week, aim to do two to four sets each of multiple exercises that train each muscle and its different functions/movements (discussed in an upcoming section).

However, your body doesn't care what exercises you perform; it cares about the mechanical tension on a specific muscle. The exercise you use is just a means of providing mechanical tension in a muscle.

So, instead of looking at an exercise and determining the number of sets to do, you should look at the muscles the exercise works and the number of sets it adds to each muscle.

Using the squat as an example, if you were to do 3 sets of squats, you would count 3 sets for the quadriceps, 3 sets for the glutes, and possibly 3 sets for your erector spinae (lower-back muscles).

So, if your workout called for 9 sets of quadriceps exercises in that specific training session, you would need 6 more sets of quadriceps exercises. This could be 3 sets of leg extensions and 3 sets of lunges. So, in total, you would complete 9 sets for the quadriceps by doing 3 sets of squats, 3 sets of leg extensions, and 3 sets of lunges.

I realize that knowing which exercises train which muscles can be difficult, but we will break them down in an upcoming section. All you need to know is that you are performing a set per muscle, not per exercise.

Next, it should be clear that men new to strength training will do considerably fewer sets than men who are more experienced. If you're a beginner at strength training, you'll need to start at the lower recommended number of sets (that's 12 total sets per muscle per week) and slowly build up until your body can handle more sets.

Since this can be difficult for new trainees to implement, I have included a program to guide you, starting at 12 sets per muscle.

The more advanced you are, the more sets your body can handle and the higher your optimal weekly set number will be. This is because your body will be more resistant to muscle damage and fatigue, and will recover faster from a given workout.

So, after about three months of consistent, hard training, you should be able to increase your total number of sets per muscle to 14, and then to 16 after another three months or so.

Each person has an optimum training volume, compared to which doing less or more results in worse results. Our goal is to ensure that you perform enough sets per muscle group to stimulate but not annihilate your muscles. With the heaviness of the weights you'll be lifting, you won't need an infinite number of sets to build muscle. In fact, by doing more than this, you will get worse results, not better.

DO 6 TO 8 AND 12 TO 15 REPS

To be able to progressively overload, build strength, prevent injuries, and maximize your muscle-building potential, you will do 6 to 8 reps per set for compound exercises and 12 to 15 reps per set for isolation exercises.

In fitness circles, there is a common myth that refuses to die out, no matter how many studies disprove it: the myth of the "hypertrophy zone."

The idea behind it is that there is an optimal zone for the number of reps you should perform to build muscle. If you do fewer reps, the thinking goes, you are only building strength; if you do more, you are only building endurance.

While it might sound convincing, research has disproved this hypertrophy zone myth. In fact, all the studies that have been done on this topic up to this point have confirmed that a given volume of low reps per set is just as effective for muscle growth as that volume in the form of higher reps per set.

For example, one study discovered that performing 4 sets of 3 to 5 reps produces the same muscle-growth results as performing 3 sets of 9 to 11 reps.[1]

However, the problem we run into is the ability to keep progressing and building muscle through increasing strength. If you are training with really high reps (say, 20 to 30), you will build muscle in the short term, but your strength won't increase much.

Also, doing high-rep work can be very fatiguing for your body. It takes a solid cardiovascular system to last that long, and it can cause muscle and neuromuscular fatigue. This can lead to feeling drained and using poor technique, inevitably leading to less weight lifted in the subsequent sets. If you've ever done 20 reps of heavy squats to the point where you couldn't complete another rep, you know exactly what I'm talking about.

So, too light a weight is fatiguing and difficult to build consistent strength with.

On the other hand, very heavy weights, in the 1-to-5-rep range, will significantly improve your strength—but the volume and time of tension on your muscles aren't enough to maximize muscle building.

Also, lifting very heavy weights requires perfect technique and strong bones, tendons, and ligaments, or you are more likely to get injured.

So, to progress with strength gains while building muscle, you will perform your compound exercises with a rep range of 6 to 8 reps.

Compound exercises—those that use multiple joints in unison—are able to handle and move more weight than isolation (or single-joint) exercises. Compound and isolation exercises are discussed in an upcoming section.

As for whether you should use 6, 7, or 8 reps, beginners should use the higher rep number and lighter weight, i.e., 8 reps. Then, after two to three months of training, decrease the number of reps and increase the weight.

If you have been weight lifting for at least a few months and your technique is solid, start at the lower reps and heavier weight, i.e., 6 reps.

The 6 to 8 reps should be heavy but not too heavy. However, this might be heavier than you are used to, so take your time perfecting your weight-lifting technique, give yourself enough rest, and push yourself to lift as much weight as possible for the main compound exercises.

After a few weeks of adjusting to this new rep scheme, you'll realize just how enjoyable lifting heavy weights and being incredibly strong can be.

When it comes to isolation (or single-joint) exercises, you will need to use lighter weights, which will naturally increase the number of reps you can perform. Isolation exercises place more stress on a single joint and, if done with a heavy weight, are more likely to cause injuries.

So, you will increase your rep range to 12 to 15 reps for isolation exercises.

Current trainees will start at 12 reps. Novices will begin with 15 reps and work down to 12 reps over time.

This is a fairly high rep range, but if you push yourself on the key compound exercises discussed later, these isolation exercises will benefit from a higher rep range.

These two rep ranges will maximize the amount of muscle you can build, increase your strength, minimize fatigue, and help prevent unnecessary injuries.

However, you need to use a heavy enough weight that you can do only the recommended number of reps on the first set of an exercise. If your weight is too light or too heavy and you don't hit the rep number you should be hitting on that first set, you will need to make adjustments (coming up).

For example, suppose a workout has a prescribed intensity of 8 reps for the first set of an exercise. In that case, you should be lifting the maximum amount of weight you can to complete only those 8 reps—no more, no less.

In a future workout, if you can complete 1 more repetition with that same weight, then that maximum weight you could do for 8 reps becomes the maximum weight you can lift for 9 reps. So, you should increase the weight to ensure that you're able to complete a maximum of only 8 reps again.

If you kept the same weight and did only 8 reps when you could have performed 9, that workout might be submaximal. In other words, if you keep training with your former 8-rep-max (8RM) weight instead of your current 8RM, each workout will not stimulate your muscles enough, and your workouts will become too submaximal, which means little to no results.

For now, simply adjusting weight as needed will suffice. In the next chapter, we'll discuss the perfect method for ensuring that you progress properly in every session.

STAY 1 REP AWAY FROM FAILURE

When using the rep scheme we've just discussed, you want to complete all the reps (either 6 to 8 or 12 to 15) on the first set but not be able to perform another rep if you were to try. This keeps you 1 repetition away from failure, or from using lousy technique to get the weight up.

If you scroll through social media, follow fitness blogs, or have spent any time in the gym, you've probably heard that "you need to go to failure" or that you need to work as hard as you can until "your muscles are completely dead."

I'm sure you've been in the gym and seen some bros attempting 1 final rep to look tough and not have the weight collapse on top of them, so they do everything in their power to complete it—including throwing technique out the window.

This is the old-school way of thinking, where hard work is thought to beat smart work. It is perpetuated by people in the gym who have no idea what they're talking about, have short careers, have had many lifting injuries, or just want to sound tough.

Logically, it might make sense that getting 1 more rep in by going to complete failure on a lift will mean more mechanical tension on a muscle. But while this might be true, you must remember that building muscles is a balancing act. Going to complete failure on one exercise or set can throw off your whole training session and even future training sessions.

Now, I want you to understand that fatigue can be good, but too much of it is bad.

You need to work your muscles enough to stress all your muscle fibers. To do this, you need to work close to fatigue so that they all come into effect. If you are too far away from fatigue or failure, some of the larger fibers won't receive enough tension.

However, once you have told a specific muscle that it needs to grow through enough volume, reps, work, intensity, and sets, continuing to place stress on that muscle can have a detrimental effect.

So, instead of going to technical failure on every single set, leaving a rep or two in the tank is far better.

And don't worry; research has conclusively shown that as long as you are within a few reps of failure, you will experience the same muscle growth as you would by going to complete failure.[2]

Not pushing yourself to failure will also allow you not to have to rely on a spotter to help you finish the last few reps that would crush you otherwise. Instead, you can work out alone without any distractions, without worrying that you won't be able to get the final rep off your chest or back without injuring yourself or looking like a fool.

By staying 1 rep away from failure, or more specifically, proper-technique failure, you will get all the benefits without any of the possible side effects that could end your strength-training career.

TRAIN EACH MUSCLE TWICE A WEEK

Based on the number of recommended sets and the time it takes for muscles to recover fully, you will have a muscle-training frequency of at least twice per week.

The truth is, your muscles don't care how often you're in the gym or what your training split is. They only react to how often and how much they experience high mechanical tension. It would be awesome if the time course of muscle growth were exactly a week long, but that just isn't true.

Training frequency isn't all that important if you can perform the same amount of work in one workout as you can in multiple workouts.

However, you can stimulate only so much muscle growth in one workout. The body's adaptive capacity is limited.

Once you have maximized your body's adaptive capacity, doing 10 more exercises to train that muscle will only lead to excess fatigue, muscle damage, and digging yourself into a deeper recovery hole to climb out of.

There's also a limit to the amount of quality work you can do in a session. As your workout progresses, your body will be able to produce less and less force and, in turn, less and less mechanical tension. You will also get mentally fatigued, and your motivation to train hard will dwindle, no matter how much pre-workout powder you chug down.

It is beneficial to increase your training frequency per muscle to combat this. When you split up a given number of exercises or sets across more sessions, you'll perform more work because you'll be less fatigued on average.

For example, do you think you could complete more total repetitions and weight by doing five exercises for one muscle in a single workout or by doing those same exercises over five days and five workouts?

So, when you train close to failure, increasing a muscle's training frequency almost always increases the number of reps and the weight you can lift for each exercise.[3]

For this reason, you will train each muscle at least twice a week—using the same numbers of sets we just discussed.

Notice that I said "at least" twice a week. You can train each muscle every day or every other day, as long as the total number of sets per muscle per week remains the same. How you choose to split the muscles up isn't important to consider at this juncture.

TAKE AT LEAST ONE DAY OFF PER WEEK

Based on the number of sets you are doing and the amount of weight you're lifting, your muscles might be able to recover without taking a single day off each week. This would be those people you see on social media who think it's better to take #nodaysoff than to let their bodies recover and rebuild.

The problem with this mentality is that, although your muscles might be able to recover, you're not stressing only your muscles when you lift heavy weights. Multiple other systems in your body don't recover as quickly as your muscles.

Having at least one day away from the gym and away from any intense exercise helps your other body tissues recover, repair, and become more resistant to damage.

Your bones, tendons, and ligaments take much longer to heal from heavy weight lifting than your muscles do, so training intensely with zero rest days will slowly overtrain them until you become injured.

Along with your body tissue, your hormones and nervous system need time to recover. If you don't allow both of these systems time to adapt and recover, you can have dwindling motivation, poor muscle and nerve learning and firing, irritability, and just poor muscle growth.

Altogether, these are signs of overtraining syndrome. Overtraining has a lot of adverse effects that are easy to avoid if you (1) stick to the correct numbers of sets we talked about and (2) take at least one day off from exercise each week.

The "work harder, not smarter" mentality is nothing new. But a happy balance of both is the best way to build muscle while ensuring longevity in the gym.

A day or two off will prevent injuries and overtraining and allow you to build more muscle by giving your muscles a bit of extra time to grow. In fact, novice and intermediate lifters have been shown to continue to grow muscles for 24 to 72 hours after a workout.

CHAPTER 17

HOW TO CONSISTENTLY BUILD MORE MUSCLE AND STRENGTH

As I said earlier in the book, if you're not getting stronger, you're more than likely not getting bigger. Similarly, I stated that in this program, you will optimize every training variable to increase your strength in one way or another.

In this chapter, we will add in the training variables that will help you consistently perform as many reps as possible with as much weight as possible. You will maintain the same intensity—6 to 8 or 12 to 15 reps—but you'll be able to progressively increase the amount of weight you can use when completing those reps.

To do this properly, you will take a strategic approach to progression by applying the best methods for progressive overload, the optimal rest periods between sets, the correct lifting tempo, and the correct way to prepare for heavy lifting.

All of these training variables work synergistically to ensure that you get consistent and measurable improvements in your strength, muscle growth, or both.

However, this will require more structure and effort, since you'll need to program for future sessions, understand what's working and what needs to be adjusted, and be competent in the gym.

For proper progression to work, you need to know how to track your progress and improve your sleep, stress levels, diet, and routine.

And if you do not have a solid technique and a feel for the movement patterns, you don't understand how to navigate weight and rep adjustments, or you're not willing to keep track of the weights you're using from session to session, then the variables in this chapter are just words on a page.

But if you are ready to put in the effort, you can get incredible, consistent results just by implementing the variables discussed below.

Let's get into the best way to make consistent strength gains and continue to progress as efficiently as possible.

REST 2 TO 4 OR 1 TO 2 MINUTES BETWEEN SETS

Your rest periods will be 2 to 4 minutes for heavy compound exercises and between 1 and 2 minutes for isolation exercises. This should be long enough to let your muscles recover adequately to do as many repetitions as possible on the next set. It should also be enough so that you don't have trouble breathing or feel mentally drained.

Old-school bodybuilders and bro-science weight lifters have preached the need for short rest periods between sets. The old-school goal was to work as hard as possible, maximize the muscle pump, and ensure that you worked your muscles until they were completely drained—the misguided thought being that the burn lets you know it's working.

As we've discussed, your goal isn't to completely burn out your muscles and create as large a pump as possible. Instead, your goal is to create as much muscle as possible to create the best physique possible. Simple as that.

The goal, then, is to lift as much weight as possible for as long as possible, i.e., the total number of reps completed with a specific weight.

It should be relatively easy to understand that if you give your muscles more rest between sets, they will be able to lift heavier weights for more repetitions. This might be hard to believe, as a lot of the information you hear says that longer rest periods help with strength but not with building muscle, but many studies have disproven this.

For example, one large and highly regarded study found far greater muscle growth and strength in a training program with a 2.5-minute rest versus a 1-minute rest.[1] Many studies have conclusively backed this finding.

Ideally, you should rest between your working sets until your muscles have recovered enough to perform optimally and you aren't struggling to breathe.

For heavy compound exercises like squats, the length of your rest period can go up to 3 to 4 minutes or more before you can lift enough weight for maximal reps.

However, most people don't like to (or simply don't have the time to) rest this long. Resting 3 to 4 minutes or more between your sets might allow you to perform more repetitions throughout the whole workout, but if you get bored and start to lose motivation because you're spending your rest time scrolling through social media or just counting down the seconds, you're not going to enjoy the workout or be able to keep it up for the long term.

So, look to bridge the gap between the benefits of long rest periods for muscle building and the benefits of short rest periods to limit time in the gym and prevent boredom.

With these things in mind, I suggest a rest period of 2 to 4 minutes between sets of heavy compound exercises like the squat, bench press, shoulder press, etc. Two minutes of rest is the bare minimum amount of time you should give yourself between sets. It's long enough to complete most of your recovery and catch your breath, but it's also short enough to avoid doom-scrolling on social media.

At any time, you can easily bump the rest periods up to 3 to 4 minutes or more for strenuous exercises, or if you're having trouble catching your breath on an off day.

On the other hand, isolation exercises allow shorter rest periods between working sets. Since isolation exercises are less technically difficult and often train much smaller muscles, you can get away with a rest period of 1 to 2 minutes.

Personally, it's hard for me to convince myself to rest longer than 2 minutes on exercises like the triceps extension when I feel fully recovered and am so close to finishing my workout.

KEEP A STEADY LIFTING TEMPO

Do your exercises at a steady, moderate, and coordinated pace. Don't try to move the weight quickly, or to intentionally slow it down.

The classic recommendation—that you should perform your reps at a 1-1-1 pace (1 second per phase of the movement), or that you need to do them slowly to increase time under tension—is either misguided or meant only for beginners.

The thought behind the 1-1-1 pace or any other variation is that you'll prevent using momentum while moving the weight, decrease the potential for injury, and work your concentric, isometric, and eccentric muscle actions.

As for time under tension, the idea is correct, but the execution behind it is incorrect. You can lift for the same amount of time by moving the weight more slowly or by doing more reps. However, by moving it slowly, you will have to use less weight, and you will complete fewer reps.

The goal with rep speed is to increase the total amount of work you do by completing as many reps as possible with as much weight as possible, while also getting the benefits of both active and passive tension.

There is no need to make this topic complicated or add fanciness to simplicity. When doing a rep, simply move the weight at a comfortable pace that allows you to maintain tension in your muscles, increase the number of reps you do, and maintain proper technique and control over the weight.

Most people will naturally perform a 1-0.5-1-0.5 rep tempo, meaning they take a beat for the first movement, take a split second for transitioning in the middle of the rep, complete the second half of the movement at a steady pace similar to the first part of the movement, and take a brief pause to take in some air and reset mentally and physically before beginning the movement again.

The numbers don't represent exact seconds but similar time frames or beats per movement based on the exercise, trainee experience, and anatomy.

No matter what, try to keep your pace consistent day in and day out to help determine whether you are actually improving. You do not need to (or even necessarily want to) count your rep speed, as this often leads to improper technique and inconsistency.

PROGRESS IN WEIGHT USING MICROLOADING

The best way to progress in your program is to simply add weight. You do the same program and reps but with more weight. If you are able to hit the prescribed reps, you will add weight to the exercise in the next training session and repeat.

Remember, if you're not getting stronger, you're probably not getting bigger or causing muscle growth. This is important because the real results don't come from the weight you start with or the number of repetitions you can complete with that weight. Instead, your results come from placing your body under new stress, i.e., progressing.

You also need to remember that you're using a program, not a random plan, with a specific rep target and prescribed weight progression model to give you consistent improvement.

As we discussed earlier, there are two ways to increase the mechanical tension you place on your body to keep producing more muscle:

1.   Increase the number of repetitions using the same weight.

2.   Increase the weight and perform the same number of repetitions.

To keep your program consistent and stay within the optimal rep range while also getting incredibly strong, you will keep your rep target the same and gradually increase the weight you use.

So, as soon as you hit the correct number of reps for a given weight on your first hard set, you will increase the weight in the next training session that uses the same exercise.

You do not need to care how many reps you complete on your following sets, since your first set already proved that you are progressing properly and getting stronger. The remaining sets are to provide enough volume for growth.

When you add weight, your goal for your next workout is to reach your prescribed rep target. To be able to do this and stay consistent, you should increase the weight by the smallest possible increment that you have. This is called microloading and is crucial for avoiding yo-yoing in strength and progression.

At most gyms, the lowest increment is 2.5 pounds for barbell exercises (5 pounds total) and 5 pounds per dumbbell (10 pounds total).

To help you understand this better, let's look at an example.

If you are doing the bench press and your workout calls for 6 reps at 200 pounds, you should be lifting the maximum amount of weight you can to complete only those 6 reps—staying 1 or 2 reps away from technical failure. Basically, if you went for another rep, you would have to use bad technique or would be unable to complete the rep.

Your program has you doing 4 sets of bench presses with a rep target of 6 and a weight increment of 5 pounds (2.5 pounds on each side of the barbell).

In the last session, you did 200 pounds x 6, 5, 4, 4 reps. Since we only care about the reps on the first set, you are microloading and progressing in this next session.

In this session, your target would then be 205 pounds for 6 reps (with perfect form, of course). This time you get 205 pounds x 6, 4, 4, 3 reps. In your upcoming session for the bench press, you will increase the weight again, to 210 pounds x 6 reps.

If you cannot perform enough reps to hit your normal rep target, say 6 in the example, then you are not progressing properly and something needs to be adjusted.

If you have an optimized program with a good routine and diet, the only time you should not be able to increase the weight you are lifting consistently—and therefore your strength—is when you reach the elite level and are near your genetic potential, or the minimum weight jump is too great for the specific exercise.

This is proper weight progression. However, no matter how good your diet and program are, there will be times when you aren't able to increase the weight and hit the correct number of repetitions.

DELOAD UPON PROGRESSION FAILURE

Not progressing with each workout session is normal. It happens often, so it's important to know how to avoid letting one missed rep target become a major problem.

If you can't hit your rep target on your first working set, you should deload your weight. This means that you lower the weight back to your previous workout session's weight.

You then perform your remaining sets as you normally would.

The next workout after you fail at a weight, you will drop back down to the previous weight you were using before the failure. This time, you'll be aiming to add another rep to your previous rep progression.

Once you can increase your reps by 1 or 2 more on your first hard set, you can attempt to raise your resistance and weight in the training session after.

Here is an example:

- You are doing 4 sets of bench presses with a rep target of 6 and a weight increment of 5 pounds. In the first session, you did 200 pounds x 6, 5, 4, 4 reps; but again, we only care about that first set.

- In bench press workout number two, you increased the weight to 205 pounds and your target was 6 reps, but you were able to complete only 5 on your first set.

- So, you deload the weight back down to 200 pounds and finish your remaining 3 sets without counting reps, because they don't matter.

- In bench-press workout number three, you drop back down to 200 pounds. You remain at this weight until you can complete 7 reps—1 more than you could do previously. For this workout, your reps go like this: 200 pounds x 7, 5, 5, 4 reps.

- In bench-press workout number four, you can increase the weight to 205 pounds again and attempt to hit 6 reps. If you hit 6 reps, you progress to 210 pounds in workout number five. But if you miss the 6 reps again in workout four, you deload your weight and increase your rep progression by 1 more. This would be 8 reps at 200 pounds instead of 7 reps.

- Repeat this process of rep progression, weight progression, and deloading.

Rep progression is also important to consider if the weight increase at one time is too great due to equipment, not poor progression. You're still getting stronger—just not as quickly as the increments of weight you have available.

For instance, if you are doing single-arm curls with a 25-pound dumbbell and the next dumbbell available is 30 pounds, this is an increase of 20%. But the standard strength increase is only 1%–2.5%. This scenario makes microloading impossible.

When this happens, you have two options:

- Increase the weight and slowly increase the repetitions until you reach the desired rep target. For example, you could go from 20 pounds x 12 to 25 pounds x 4 reps, then 5 reps the next workout, etc., until you reach 25 pounds x 12 reps, and then you go up to 30 pounds.

- Increase repetitions until you are more readily able to increase the weight. For example, you could go from 20 pounds x 12 to 20 pounds x 13, then 14 reps the next workout, etc., until you can increase the weight comfortably to 25 pounds x 8 to 12 reps.

As you can see, progressing in strength is very important. It truly is what separates people with amazing bodies from those who are stuck in the same bodies they've been trying to transform for years.

WARM UP FOR EACH TRAINING SESSION

Start every session with 5 to 15 minutes of light cardio followed by 1 to 3 increasingly heavier warm-up sets, using a full range of motion, of the first exercise for each muscle group you are training in that session (when you get to that exercise in your program).

This might have you doubting whether this is enough or too much, because when it comes to warming up, there are two trains of thought. Either it is vital and you need to do everything in your power to get a good warm-up, or you don't need to warm up at all. Science lies somewhere in the middle.

The goal of warming up for strength training is simple: to warm your body enough to lift heavy weights and prevent injury. To do this, you need to increase your body's internal temperature and then prepare the specific muscles you plan to train.

In general, you can increase your body temperature by simply performing low-intensity cardio or even walking around with sweats on. During this process, as the name suggests, your body temperature literally rises, or warms up.

Research has shown that for warming up, 15 minutes of low-intensity cardio is more beneficial than only 5 minutes of high-intensity cardio.[2]

Next, to prepare the muscles you're going to train, you want to work them through the range of motion they are about to undergo and get them used to the movements they'll perform. To accomplish this, perform with low intensity the exact weight-lifting movement you are going to do.

Start every exercise with at least one warm-up set to prepare your muscles, tendons, joints, and nerves for more weight. Heavy exercises like squats, bench presses, and deadlifts may call for more warm-up sets with increasing intensity.

So, to prepare your body for an intense training session, you need a brief warm-up until you are sufficiently warmed. Typically, this means you start to break a sweat.

You do not need to time your warm-ups or hit a certain number. If you are cold or not mentally prepared to lift heavy weights, keep warming up. If, after 5 minutes, you are warm, sweating, and ready to go, get going on your light warm-up sets.

Most often, about 10 minutes of light cardio is the sweet spot. You can do this by walking on a treadmill, rowing, or cycling if you're at the gym.

Remember, fatigue has a detrimental effect on building muscles, so you're not there to wear yourself out before your actual training session begins. Instead, you're doing this to prepare for your training session.

When it comes to your warm-up sets, 2 or 3 for the first exercise for a specific muscle group is ideal. Then 1 for every remaining exercise is the maximum needed.

Do about 30%–50% of your working weight, then 50%–80%, then 80%–100% with the same number of reps that your program calls for for that specific exercise. Again, concentrate on technique and range of motion.

Don't overthink it. If you need more, do more. Just make sure you do something.

As a note, if you warm up and your muscles or joints still ache, you might need to adjust your technique or volume/sets. These two major factors will cause injuries—one from excessive strain on a joint and the other from overtraining.

This is different from just being sore. Being sore is not the enemy, but it also isn't the goal—it simply happens like smoke from a campfire. You can train while sore with no adverse effects, but being sore is not a sign of a good workout or more muscle growth.

STRETCH AS NEEDED, EXCEPT AROUND TRAINING

In general, stretching just makes you better at stretching. You're not lengthening your muscles or altering your joints, tendons, or ligaments in any way.

Instead, by stretching, you're telling your body that a specific range of motion is okay and won't hurt you. Your nerves relax, which lets you do that stretch or range of motion without sending pain signals to your brain.

Then, the next time you perform that same stretch, your body will know that it won't get injured at that joint and muscle length, so it will allow you to stretch even further.

This is similar to the neuromuscular changes that your body goes through when you begin lifting weights. When you lift weights, your neuromuscular system adapts to help you lift more. Likewise, when you stretch, your neuromuscular system adapts to help you stretch more.

As strength trainers, our only goal is to have a full range of motion in our exercises. These are basically sport-specific movements. So we have a reason for our flexibility.

So, what is the easiest way to increase your range of motion and improve your neural tolerance?

Perform the movements! During your warm-up sets, do your movements and exercises and consciously try to increase your range of motion. This is similar to doing dynamic sport-specific stretching, like leg swings before running.

It's also worth noting that static stretching has been shown to be detrimental to power, strength, and muscle growth, especially when performed before working out. This is because you're telling your muscles to relax instead of preparing them for work.[3]

When it comes to stretching during a warm-up, all you have to do is perform some dynamic stretching of the muscles and joints you will use and then do some warm-up sets of the exercise you'll be doing. These could be shoulder rolls, toe touches, or body-weight squats. If you feel you need to stretch, just do it. But don't hold your stretches in a static position.

If you enjoy stretching or taking a yoga class every so often, then go ahead. Just try to space your stretching as far away from your strength training as possible.

SECRET 6

-

YOUR TRAINABLE MUSCLES, WHAT THEY DO, AND THE BEST EXERCISES FOR DEVELOPING THEM

CHAPTER 18

SELECTING THE BEST STRENGTH-TRAINING EXERCISES

Each of your skeletal muscles performs a specific function that helps you complete a movement pattern, like walking, jumping, twisting, or lifting and moving objects.

Strength-training exercises are the means by which force is transferred to specific muscle functions to make them work harder to complete a specific movement pattern. They train your muscles by training the function of a muscle.

Their job is not to help you lift as much weight as possible to impress your friends or to make you do a lot of unnecessary and fancy movements to burn calories, make you breathe hard, or look athletic. Each exercise in your program should be chosen to help you grow a specific muscle by placing the right amount of stress over all of its muscle fibers. In other words, each exercise has a purpose. So, it's important to know how each muscle moves your body, that is, how it functions, and which exercises allow you to train that movement.

Just as importantly, you need to know the best exercises to train the different muscles within the muscle group and how many different exercises, also known as exercise variety or exercise variations, are needed to develop the whole muscle group.

EXERCISE SELECTION AND VARIATION

For all of a muscle's fibers to be stimulated, the number of exercises you do should be proportional to the number of functions the muscle performs, but you probably don't need more variety than that.

With proper programming, in which you lift heavy weights to near technical failure, your body will call upon as many muscle fibers as it can to help perform the movement pattern.

With the correct intensity and volume, you can stress nearly all of the muscle fibers that help with a movement pattern without needing 10 slightly different exercises for that same muscle.

So, when it comes to exercise variety and the number of exercises for a muscle and muscle group, combined with the volume, intensity, and proximity to failure, it is more beneficial to use only a few select exercises to train each muscle's major functions.

Rather than stressing about trying to train every single fiber of every muscle from every angle, keep your attention on the progression of a selection of key exercises.

THE BEST TYPES OF STRENGTH-TRAINING EXERCISES

There is no strength-training exercise in the world that can't be replaced. Still, some exercises are better suited for building awesome-looking and functionally strong muscles than others.

The exercises that will give you the biggest bang for your buck are (1) free-weight (2) compound exercises that allow you to move through (3) a full range of motion while maintaining (4) constant tension through (5) dynamic muscle contractions.

Free Weights

Compared with machines, free weights, such as barbells and dumbbells, result in significantly greater muscle growth and strength development, better improvements in balance, and fewer injuries, because free weights allow greater freedom of movement instead of being stuck to a fixed movement pattern.[1]

Compound Movements

Compound exercises, which call on multiple muscles to cause movement using multiple joints, allow you to lift more weight, develop more strength, provide more potential for muscle growth, train multiple muscles simultaneously, burn more calories, improve coordination, and save time.[2]

Isolation exercises, which cause movement of a single joint, are generally reserved for "filling in the gaps" for each muscle group.

Even when muscle activation is the same, compound exercises are generally more efficient because they train multiple muscles at the same time.

Maximal Range of Motion

Exercises that allow for a larger range of motion build more muscle and strength, improve flexibility, ensure that the whole muscle is stressed (since some muscles aren't activated or stressed until the end of a movement), and avoid putting too much stress on muscles, joints, bones, tendons, and cartilage, which can cause injuries. These exercises also develop the best-operating, best-looking, and best-shaped muscles.[3]

That being said, your range of motion is determined by your individual joints, muscles, and flexibility, not by the maximal range of motion that an exercise allows or by an arbitrary point in space. For example, your glutes and quads don't reach a full range of motion when you do a deadlift, but the floor and the arbitrary size of the weight plates prevent further movement. Similarly, a full squat should be as deep as you are able to go without pain and while maintaining good form. The common recommendation of squatting until the fronts of your thighs are parallel to the floor is nothing more than a way to get half-squatting gym-bros to finally attempt deeper squats.

Dynamic Muscle Actions and Constant Tension

When doing a repetition, your muscles should maintain tension by continuously moving the weight through a concentric, or positive, muscle action, with the muscle contracting and shortening, immediately followed by an eccentric, or negative, muscle action, with the muscle lengthening under tension. This should be immediately followed by another concentric muscle action, i.e., the next repetition.[4]

An isometric contraction, in which the muscles have tension but aren't moving, will occur naturally when transitioning between concentric and eccentric muscle actions, but it should be kept as brief as possible. And if muscle tension is lost or an exercise doesn't complete dynamic muscle actions, then it is not ideal.

CHAPTER 19

THE FIVE KEY EXERCISES FOR ALL-AROUND MUSCLE

Research has shown that an exercise improves strength the most when performed first in a training session.[1] This correlates to more muscle growth for the muscles that the exercise trains.

So, you should prioritize exercises that you would like to get stronger in and exercises that train the muscles you want or need to develop by doing them first or very early in a training session.

However, you need to place heavy, technically difficult, compound exercises, which primarily train larger muscle groups, before easier-to-perform isolation exercises and those that train a smaller muscle group, especially if they train the same muscle.

Basically, for the more difficult exercises that will build more muscle, you want to be mentally fresh and able to give all your effort while maintaining perfect technique.

Compound exercises that train a large muscle group, like your lats, pecs, deltoids, or thighs, will also use smaller muscle groups to help complete the exercise. So, if you work a smaller muscle group first, you create a weak link in the chain.

For instance, back exercises often use the biceps; chest and shoulder moves often call on the triceps; and quad and hamstring exercises frequently involve the glutes and lower back.

To maximize your results, you will be prioritizing five key exercises. These moves will give you the most bang for your buck when it comes to developing the exact muscles that are desired most.

Each of these five priority exercises incorporates the proper muscle functions of your major muscles while also allowing you to move a significant amount of weight to build impressive all-around strength.

To build a broad and square upper body with a beautiful taper, you will concentrate your efforts on three primary exercises—the pull-up, the flat bench press, and the seated dumbbell shoulder press.

These three exercises will build your arms, shoulders, back, and chest, creating a well-balanced, strong, and aesthetically pleasing upper body that will flow nicely into your midsection and lower body.

To target your lower body, you will perform the barbell back squat and the barbell Romanian deadlift, or RDL.

Squats will develop your quadriceps, or quads, on the front of your thighs. Romanian deadlifts will develop your hamstrings, on the back of your thighs. Both exercises will also develop your glutes simultaneously.

These two exercises by themselves can give you enough muscle to create legs that are muscular and proportional to your upper body.

Again, the goal is to use these five exercises as your go-to moves when starting a training session and to ensure that you give as much effort as possible to each of these exercises.

If you train hard with these five exercises, progress in weight properly, and ensure that you have perfect technique, I promise you that you will build an amazing body.

Just throw in some complementary exercises to target the few remaining muscles and reach the optimal weekly sets, and you will be on your way to intense but short workouts that will give you the best body of your life.

Quick Note on Technique

It's very important that you do each of these five exercises (and all other exercises) correctly. If I could restart my strength-training journey, the first thing I would do is learn and perfect the proper techniques.

Having the correct hand and foot placement, range of motion, repetition speed, and more takes time to learn and implement. But doing an exercise with proper form, even if you have to lower the weight to get it correct, will build more strength, reduce injuries from excess strain on joints, bones, tendons, and ligaments, and build more functional and aesthetic muscle over the long term.

Research on learning proper technique has shown that trying to get every single detail correct and going through each step one at a time is actually detrimental to the learning process. Instead, you should learn what the exercise should look like and the correct starting and finishing positions. Then concentrate on only a few internal cues, like "prevent knees from caving in" on the squat or "don't flare your elbows" when bench pressing. This will allow you to let your body move more naturally.

To learn the proper techniques, look for videos on YouTube or Google from professional educators such as Menno Henselmans and Mark Rippetoe (rather than professional bodybuilders or fitness influencers). You can also use professional resources such as exrx.net/lists/directory.

EXERCISE #1: PULL-UP

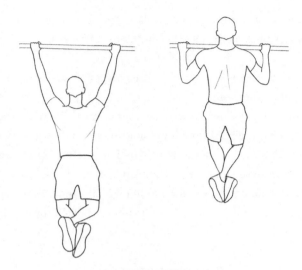

Building a strong back can have a real impact on how your body looks and functions. The back should be wide and thick, so it tapers nicely down to a lean waist, pulls your shoulders back, and ties in your upper body and lower body beautifully.

In order to create a strong and aesthetically pleasing back, you will prioritize the pull-up. This move will fully train your latissimus dorsi, middle and lower trapezius, and biceps.

When well developed, the latissimus dorsi, commonly known as the lats, create the appearance of "wings" that can be seen from the front, beneath your armpits.

Most exercises for working your back muscles do a mediocre job of developing the lats because they don't provide a full range of motion.

In the pull-up movement, the lats help to pull your arm from above your head to in front of your body and/or to the side of your body. This is almost 180 degrees of motion.

If you have a weight belt—where you attach weight to a metal chain and then place a belt around your hips and waist for added resistance—and can do enough pull-ups, I highly recommend that you prioritize the wide-grip weighted pull-up to train your lats optimally. The wide grip helps train the outer fibers of your lats that provide width to your back. It will also help you create good-looking arms and develop the middlemost muscles of your back, known as the trapezius, or traps.

To train mostly the inner fibers of your lats, which are still external but are closer to your spine, you can add a reverse-grip (palms facing you) or neutral-grip (palms facing each other) weighted pull-up. If you're able, you can even rotate among the wide, reverse, and neutral grips for full development of your lats. Both the reverse and the neutral grip involve the same movement pattern—arms in front of your body—so the choice will come down to whichever one puts the least stress on your wrists and forearms. On average, the neutral-grip pull-up places far less stress on the wrists, so I typically recommend it over the reverse grip.

If you are unable to do full pull-ups, in which you start from a hanging position and bring your body all the way up until your chest touches the bar, then pull-downs might be a better option for you. Pull-downs use a cable attached to a weight stack that allows you to adjust the weight easily and to use a lower amount of weight than your body weight.

Since both the pull-up and the pull-down are able to provide tension over your lats' entire muscle length because they both allow for a full range of motion, you can use either exercise without sacrificing your gains. But I suggest relying more on movements that allow your whole body to move than on those that move the weight while most of you stays still.

EXERCISE #2: FLAT BENCH PRESS

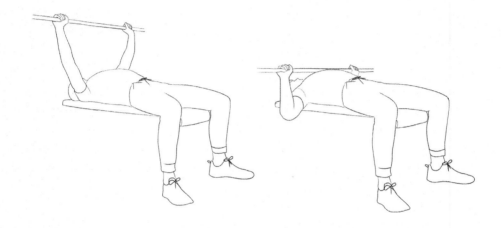

To train the front of your upper body and create a square chest, you are going to perform the flat bench press with a barbell.

The flat bench press trains the whole pectoral (chest) region, including both the upper and mid pecs, the anterior deltoids (the front of the shoulders), and the triceps (the back of the upper arm).

There is often a debate about whether it's better to do the barbell flat bench press, the barbell incline press, or the flat and incline presses with dumbbells instead of barbells. While all of these are awesome exercises, the choice will ultimately be yours based on the results you're getting, your ability to adjust the weight, and possible injuries.

When done correctly, the barbell flat bench press is a safe exercise for most people, can develop a full chest, and allows for optimal strength progression—which is why I recommend it over other bench press options.

The flat bench press works the different heads of your pectoralis major—the sternal head of the mid pec and the clavicular head of the upper pec—evenly when done from a completely flat position with minimal back arch.

However, the proper technique requires a slight arch in the back, which places your chest at a slight decline pressing angle. This slight angle can reduce the amount of upper-pec stress, which can result in less and less upper-pec growth the more you arch your back.

The incline bench press doesn't stress your upper pecs any more than a flat bench press when both are performed to technical failure. But it does place less stress on the lower heads of your pecs, so this area isn't trained optimally.

So, if you are looking to develop the whole pec, stick to the flat bench press. If you notice that you're building muscle and strength but your mid-to-lower pecs are much more developed than your upper pecs, you can switch to the incline bench press instead.

As for whether you should use a barbell or dumbbells, assuming you aren't limited by either piece of equipment, there is no wrong answer, but there are a few pros and cons of both that might sway you to prefer one over the other.

The barbell bench press is the easier exercise, since you only have to control the barbell. Barbells are also easier to microload and adjust weight on, and will develop your triceps more. However, having your hands stuck in a fixed position on a barbell can lead to discomfort in some people's shoulders and wrists.

If this is the case for you, it can be better to perform the flat bench press with dumbbells instead of a barbell. This will allow you to follow a different movement pattern and to have your wrists slightly twisted, which can relieve discomfort.

Overall, if you perform the bench-press technique correctly, progress in weight properly, and don't go to technical failure or try to squeeze in more reps by throwing technique out the window, you can have a long barbell-flat-bench-pressing career—and amazing pecs to prove it.

EXERCISE #3: SEATED DUMBBELL SHOULDER PRESS

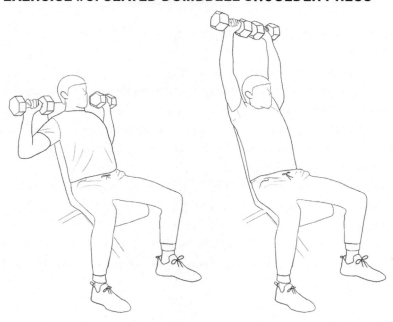

Well-developed shoulders help to give your body an amazing V taper. They provide the broad start to the V, and, when combined with nicely developed upper pecs and upper traps, they give the front of your body an aesthetic, square look that makes your waist appear skinnier.

The main muscle that creates enviable shoulders is the lateral deltoid. This is the muscle that is on the outside of the shoulder and ties directly into the arm.

We'll use the seated dumbbell shoulder press to target your lateral deltoids and develop your shoulders to their full potential while also training your triceps.

There are a few different variations of shoulder presses, and each can be beneficial, but the seated dumbbell shoulder press reigns supreme for most lifters.

The dumbbell shoulder press requires far less technique than the military press or barbell shoulder press. Even though a barbell offers added stability and facilitates microloading for proper progression, these benefits aren't worth the difficulty in performing and learning the movement.

Instead, dumbbells allow you to bring the weight directly over your head without any extra movement of your back and head. You can follow the normal motion of your shoulders and keep the weights directly above your forearms throughout the movement.

Performing the exercise seated with your back against a pad (like a chair) allows for even more stability in a movement that requires you to bring a weight directly over your head. In addition, it's far easier to get the dumbbells to and from your shoulders when you're seated than when you're standing.

Finally, since the weight is directly over your shoulders instead of in front of you, you will work the lateral deltoid more than the front deltoid, which is often overworked.

EXERCISE #4: BARBELL BACK SQUAT

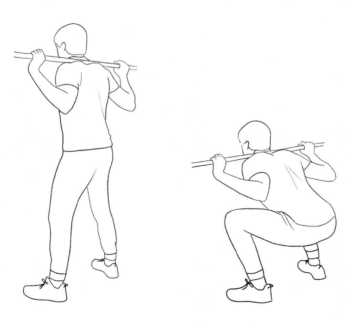

The barbell back squat is the best exercise for developing the front of your thighs, your glutes, your lower-body strength, and your core/midsection.

Of all the exercises in this chapter, the barbell back squat recruits the most muscles for completion, is the most technically difficult, and is the most strenuous.

Because the barbell back squat requires a lot of coordination, flexibility through multiple joints, variability in technique and setup, multiple muscles working in coordination, a longer distance than normal to move the weight, heavy weight directly on top of you and your spine, and more weight than most people are used to using, it provides amazing results—but it is often done incorrectly, leading to injuries.

When done correctly, the barbell back squat trains your quadriceps and glutes extensively through a full range of motion while also working your core, abs, and lower back through spinal stabilization. Keeping a tight and flexed midsection during the squat can be all the ab training you need to maintain a tight waist.

Your lower-back muscles, or spinal erectors, should form a "Christmas tree" at the end of your lats and can help keep your entire midsection tight and lean. It's very easy to tell when a weight lifter has a strong lower back from doing heavy spinal loading exercises versus when a weight lifter avoids exercises (like the squat) that require weight that loads the spine. And this latter type of lifter often experiences lower-back pain from basic lifts and from everyday life.

The main purpose of the squat in a strength-training program is to build your quads and glutes. To put it simply, squats will give you the best legs and butt possible while helping you develop a lean and muscular midsection.

For the quads, or the four muscles on the front of your leg, squats reign supreme. Naturally, the quads make up a majority of your upper-leg mass, which makes squats even more important.

However, you can't vastly change the look of your quads beyond growing the muscles. Some people's quads stretch much farther toward their knees, while others' become bulkier a few inches above the knee. In all, the end location of your muscles is based on your genetics and muscle origins.

Next, the glutes. Most men don't care too much about their glutes, but they are important muscles for function, spinal health, and aesthetics. Your glutes, specifically your gluteus maximus, work in coordination with your quads. Getting a full range of motion and providing as much mechanical tension as possible over the full muscle length by heavy squatting as deep as your body and joints allow will stretch your quads and glutes as much as possible and build the most muscle.

The standard setup for a barbell back squat is called a high bar squat, which is done with your feet about shoulder width apart.

With your feet in this stance and the bar high on your back, you will target the whole quad and glute. This is the most common back squat setup and is the most recommended for most people.

The other option is to get into a slightly wider stance. With your feet farther apart, you will place less strain on your patellar tendons and knees, which can help prevent knee pain (if you have bad knees already)—but be aware that this can place more stress on your hips.

When it comes to the squat, there are multiple reasons why I highly recommend doing barbell back squats over alternatives.

First, the back squat is easier than the front squat. Research has shown that both exercises stress your quads the same, but the back squat is easier to perform because of the placement of the weight.

Next, due to the technical difficulty and the amount of weight needed, using dumbbells or cables would be a nightmare or would just limit the amount of resistance you could use.

Overall, the back squat is a master at building muscle and strength from your midsection down to your knee caps (plus bone density and joint flexibility beyond that area).

EXERCISE #5: BARBELL ROMANIAN DEADLIFT (RDL)

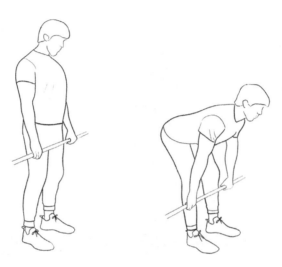

The standard deadlift or even the increasingly popular sumo deadlift is a great exercise to lift heavy weights and look strong. However, when it comes to building beautiful muscles and creating an amazing body, it isn't all it's cracked up to be. It fails to train your muscles through a full range of motion, uses only the concentric/positive muscle action, is difficult to learn and perfect, and takes an excessive amount of time and energy to set up and adjust.

Instead, we will replace the standard deadlift with a version that allows you to fill in the muscle groups that the other versions miss: the Romanian deadlift, better known as the RDL.

The RDL is a great way to train your hamstrings and glutes—in other words, the back of your lower body—through their entire range of motion.

The hamstrings work in coordination with the glutes to straighten your torso with a hinge at your hips, such as when you are bending over to pick up an object from the ground and then straightening up again. This is as long as your knees aren't bending at the same time.

When it comes to your physique, having proportionate hamstrings and quads is important. The hamstrings will help keep you from looking like your body goes straight from lats to ankles when you're wearing shorts.

Though it's natural to have larger quads than hamstrings, the problem arises when your quads take up too much of your thighs and they look disproportionate.

RDLs will also train your glutes in a similar manner to the squat. So, they will help you grow your glutes while also giving the back of your thighs great muscle development to tie into your butt and the front of your thighs.

Again, you might not care too much about growing your butt or the flow from glutes to hamstrings, but strong glute muscles are beneficial for everyday function, core stabilization, performing other lower-body movements, and preventing possible injuries due to weak glutes and/or hamstrings.

Next, if people are going to give deadlifts credit for training their traps, spinal erectors, biceps, and possibly lats (if you don't understand muscle physiology), because these muscles need to be flexed and prevent rounding of your spine, you can also add these muscles in with the muscles trained when performing the RDL.

This means that the RDL can help you maintain a strong lower, mid, and upper back when it comes to pulling your shoulders back and preventing your spine from rounding. In short, the RDL is a great exercise for developing most of your posterior.

You can perform the RDL a few different ways, but I suggest starting with the barbell. Just like with the squat and standard deadlift, the barbell allows you to move more weight due to increased stability. More weight often leads to greater tension in the muscles, greater strength, and increased muscle growth. So, as long as you can achieve a full range of motion as allowed by your hips, glutes, and hamstrings, you should use the barbell.

HOW TO CREATE A LEAN AND MUSCULAR MIDSECTION

A tight and muscular midsection that has clear separation between the muscles of the "six-pack" has long been a coveted look that a lot of men would kill for. It's the one muscle group that proves without a doubt that you're lean, work hard, and have a quality diet.

In reality, the cliché that "abs are made in the kitchen" is true. Endless crunches and the influencers' six-pack workouts are worthless because your abs won't even be seen until you are lean enough.

The real key to good-looking abs and a rocking six-pack is getting down to a low body fat percentage. To get a six-pack, you need to lose the fat that is over your abs. The ab muscles will not show or have impressive separation unless they don't have very much fat on top of them.

Men naturally store more fat around their waists than women do. This often makes it harder for men than for women to have well-defined abs.

Most males do not have visibly present abdominal muscles until they reach 10%–12% body fat or below. The closer you are to 7%–8% body fat, the more visible your six-pack and obliques will be.

Once again, you can't spot-reduce body fat, so you should spend all your time perfecting your diet and lifting heavy weights instead of trying to find the best ab workout video online.

For this reason, abdominal training should be done ad libitum, or as much and as often as needed. This will save you time and prevent you from spending excess energy trying to get a good burn in your abs without any real benefits.

A lot of men will find that by flexing their abs and tightening their core while lifting heavy weights, they will create a strong core and train their abs enough. Others will need to work on their abs a little bit more to make their muscles stand out.

I highly suggest that you don't add in any extra ab work until you get to 10%–12% body fat and can determine if you actually need it. You might realize extra crunches do nothing for you, and you can get home 10 minutes earlier from the gym.

So, add in enough abdominal work to ensure that your abs have enough development and muscle to look good, but don't spend extra time on abdominal work when you could spend it elsewhere.

The only exception to this is for beginners and those who are not able to do heavy spinal loading exercises such as squats, RDLs, pull-downs, and shoulder presses. If this applies to you, you should add in planks, both normal and side, to train your transverse abdominis.

◇◇◇

Now you have the five key exercises you should prioritize when strength training. If you take the time to practice and perfect the different techniques while ensuring proper progression with just these five exercises, you will be able to get a majority of the results you want.

These exercises should help you simplify your training program and spend less time and energy on exercises that don't help. When in doubt, just put all your effort into these five moves and add in a few complementary exercises as needed.

When combined with the rest of the knowledge from this book, these exercises will enable you to build the best-looking and best-functioning muscles.

CHAPTER 20

YOUR MUSCLES AND
HOW TO TRAIN THEM

To build all-around muscle and strength, you need to train each of the external muscles in your body with perfect technique while ensuring that your body still has great proportions.

That being said, you don't need to know every single muscle in the human body to achieve a phenomenal physique. But you do need to know the major muscles that you can train with strength training.

There are 11 major skeletal muscle groups that every strength trainer should know about. The muscles within these 11 major groups are the muscles that every person can and often should train to be able to develop a well-balanced, proportionate, injury-free, and aesthetically pleasing body.

These muscle groups are just one way among many to help classify your trainable muscles, allowing you to understand which areas of your body you need to train.

For each muscle group, I will go over the main muscles in the group with the aid of pictures. I'll describe the muscles' actions and major functions, and note how much exercise variation you need to completely develop a muscle.

Most of the top exercises for each muscle group are presented as generalized exercises because there are often many different variations on these top moves. Depending on your available workout time, equipment, anatomy, and more, you may need to use different variations of these primary exercises.

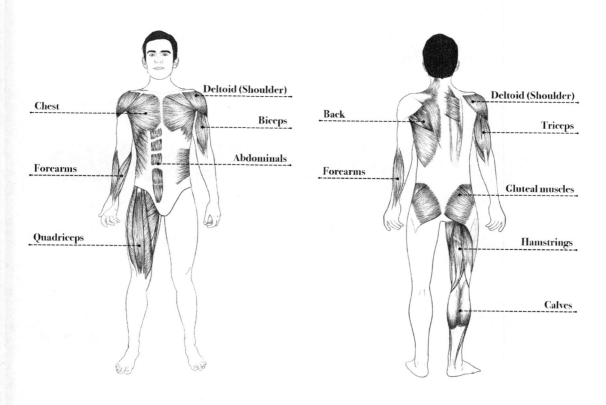

Chest

Deltoid (Shoulder)

Biceps

Abdominals

Forearms

Quadriceps

Back

Deltoid (Shoulder)

Triceps

Forearms

Gluteal muscles

Hamstrings

Calves

- Back
- Shoulders
- Chest
- Quadriceps

- Hamstrings
- Glutes
- Biceps
- Triceps

- Abdominals
- Calves
- Forearms

THE BACK

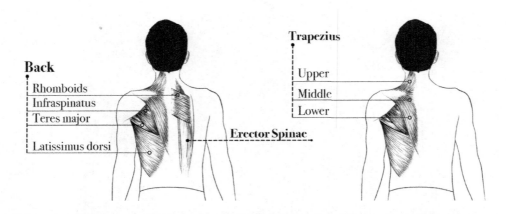

PRIMARY BACK EXERCISES

• Wide-grip pull-up/pull-down variations	• Straight-arm pull-down	• Neutral- or reverse-grip pull-up/pull-down variations
• Row variations	• Face pull	• Reverse fly
	• Shrug	

A strong back is necessary not only to help you achieve a quality physique but to help with daily lifting and carrying.

The **latissimus dorsi**, the **spinal erectors** (more specifically the erector spinae), and the **trapezius** make up most of the back.

Though visible, your infraspinatus, teres major, and teres minor cannot be specifically targeted, so they are not included as major muscles of the back. The rhomboids are not visible and do not provide a unique muscle function compared with the major trainable muscles, so they do not need to be considered when training.

The **latissimus dorsi**, often called the lats, are large, triangular muscles that extend from under the shoulders down to the lower back. The lats are the largest muscles of the upper body and therefore require the most attention. With a well-developed back, you will have strong lats that taper down to make your waist look skinnier.

The **spinal erectors** are several muscles in the lower back that help to keep the spine erect by straightening your back or preventing unwanted bending of the spine.

The **trapezius** muscles, often called the traps, are flat, triangular muscles that extend from the neck down between the shoulder blades. The traps are made up of lower, middle, and upper portions that each have different functions. The upper part of the trapezius is often included with the shoulders, as it visually connects your neck to your shoulders, but I am going to include the upper traps with the back for now. You should have muscular traps that add thickness to the middle of your back along your spine while also connecting your lats, neck, shoulders, and lower back.

Back Muscle Functions

The **lats** have two basic functions:

1. They pull the upper arms down in front of the chest, such as in a neutral- or reverse-grip pull-down motion.
2. They pull the upper arms down to the sides of the body, such as in a wide-grip pull-down motion.

The **trap** muscles have three different functions due to their different heads:

1. The upper trapezius lifts the shoulder and scapula (shoulder blade). It also helps turn the head.
2. The middle trapezius draws the scapula inward.
3. The lower trapezius pulls the scapula down toward the lower back.

The traps are the visual center of the upper back. They allow for movement in the opposite direction to the pull-down of the lats and inward movement of the shoulder blades (scapulae). The lats pull the upper arms toward the body, and the traps take over for movement of the shoulder blades inward, up, and down.

The **spinal erectors** are mostly stabilizers. They keep the body steady and erect rather than working through a full range of motion like most other muscles in the body. However, the spinal erectors do coordinate with the glutes and hamstrings for movement at the hips.

Back Training

To develop a quality back, you need to consider how each of the major muscles functions so that you can include exercises that work them.

To develop the outer lats for back width, you should include a vertical pull exercise that brings your upper arms down along your sides, like a wide-grip pull-up.

To hit the inner lats, connecting the lats to the traps, requires a vertical pull exercise that brings your arms in front of you in an arc, like a neutral- or reverse-grip pull-down.

To develop a muscular and thick middle back, you need to target all three heads of the traps. The lower head of the traps often gets worked well with vertical pulls, since the movement works in coordination with pulling your scapulae downward and together.

To develop the middle and upper heads of the traps, you can include exercises that work the traps' inward and upward scapular motion, such as reverse flies and shrugs.

If you are just starting out, a pull-down variation is a good place to start to build strength and neural connections.

THE SHOULDERS

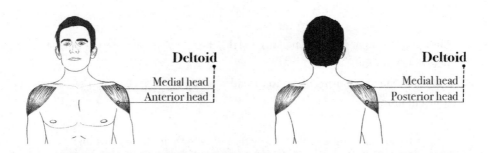

PRIMARY SHOULDER EXERCISES

- Dumbbell/barbell overhead press
- Upright row
- Shrug
- Lateral raise
- Reverse fly
- Face pull

Well-developed shoulders, scientifically called the deltoids, will create "caps" that provide the upper part of the classic V shape and flow nicely from your neck, traps, lats, and pecs to your upper arms.

Muscular shoulders make your upper body wider and, in turn, make your waist appear smaller. However, the width of your shoulders is, to a great extent, determined by your skeletal structure.

Strong shoulders are important for helping with other lifts and protecting the shoulder joints.

The deltoids make up the shoulders. They are triangular muscles that start at the collarbone and scapula and go all the way down to the upper arm.

The deltoids are composed of three heads: the **anterior (front) deltoid**, **lateral (side) deltoid**, and **posterior (rear) deltoid**. In the gym, you may hear the three heads of the deltoids called the front delt, middle delt, and rear delt.

The upper traps are often included with the shoulders. The traps help form the upper portion of your body and visually connect your shoulders to your back and neck.

Shoulder Muscle Functions

The deltoid rotates and lifts the arm. It helps to move the arm forward, backward, side to side, up, and around.

The anterior deltoid lifts the arm to the front and helps pull the arm across the chest.

1. The lateral deltoid lifts the arm to the side.
2. The posterior deltoid lifts the arm to the rear and helps pull the arm backward.

Shoulder Training

You should work to grow each of the different heads of your deltoids and create a slight separation between them.

The shoulders are worked with two basic kinds of exercises:

1. Vertical presses for size and strength
2. Arm raises to isolate specific heads

Vertical presses are multi-joint movements, so they allow you to lift more weight and are the most beneficial exercises for overall shoulder development. Vertical presses often target the lateral deltoid the most, which is the most important for developing width in your upper body.

Various types of arm raises are used to isolate the specific heads of the deltoids. They involve lifting your extended arm in an arc to the front, side, or rear.

To help target the specific muscles of the deltoid, you should do raises from different angles as needed to get the right amount of volume. This will help with separation of the three heads as well as with definition.

But front raises and extra training of the anterior deltoids are not recommended, because the front deltoid is also worked by exercises like chest presses, flies, and shoulder presses.

On the other hand, most males have underdeveloped rear delts, so you might need to give special consideration to your rear delts through exercises that pull your upper arms backward, such as face pulls and reverse flies.

THE CHEST

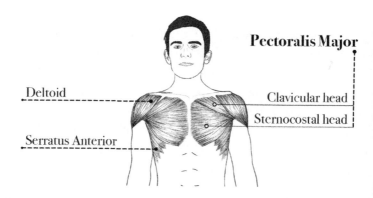

Pectoralis Major
— Clavicular head
— Sternocostal head
Deltoid
Serratus Anterior

PRIMARY CHEST EXERCISES

- Flat bench-press variations
- Incline-press variations
- Fly variations

The chest is composed of the **pectoralis major**, most often called the pectorals, or just pecs. The pectorals are attached to the rib cage and fan out across the shoulder.

Though often thought of as one muscle by most weight lifters, the pectoralis major actually consists of two parts:

1. Clavicular portion of the upper pec
2. Sternal portion of the lower and middle pec

Both attach to the sternum, in the middle of your chest and body.

To develop a quality chest, you must grow both the upper and lower/middle portions of the pecs. As with training your other muscles, you should work your pecs through a full range of motion as allowed by your joints and muscles, with minimal limitations from machines, barbells, and dumbbells.

Chest Muscle Functions

The chest muscles are involved in any hugging or horizontal pressing motion. The basic function of the pec muscles is to pull the upper arm and shoulder across the front of the body.

Chest Training

There are two basic kinds of exercises for training your chest:

1. Horizontal presses, in which the weight is pressed upward or forward from your chest
2. Flies, in which your arms are extended and drawn together across your chest

To properly train your chest, you need to develop the upper and mid/lower pecs, as well as their outer and inner sides. To do this, you need to complete bench presses from different angles and determine which angles give you the chest development and appearance you desire.

A lot of men struggle to develop their upper chest but have a well-developed middle and lower chest. When you do incline presses, most of the stress will be on your upper pecs and anterior deltoids.

The flat bench press does train your upper pecs, but with the angle of your back on the bench and to the bar or dumbbell, the upper portion might have less tension. For this reason, you probably don't need to do any lower-pec development (dips and decline bench presses) but should instead spend your efforts on incline presses and flies.

Flies are used to isolate the pecs. They are a single-joint movement that can help develop any lagging areas that are missed with presses—such as the inner pec, due to bringing your hands closer together and/or crossing over cables.

Often, the triceps and anterior deltoids fatigue before the pecs, so presses alone might not be enough to fully develop the pecs.

THE QUADRICEPS

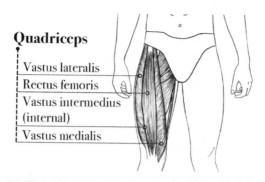

Quadriceps

Vastus lateralis
Rectus femoris
Vastus intermedius
(internal)
Vastus medialis

PRIMARY QUADRICEPS EXERCISES

• Squat	• Split squat/Bulgarian	• Leg press
• Lunge	split squat	• Leg extension

The muscles of the upper legs and thighs are the largest and strongest in your body. They are used in almost every sport and for everyday life, whether for a powerful leg drive or for endurance running.

The quadriceps, more commonly referred to as the quads, are the powerhouse of the upper legs and will take up a majority of the thigh on well-trained lifters.

The quads are the four muscles that make up the front of the thigh. They all originate from different points but converge on one common tendon.

The four muscles are the **vastus lateralis**, **vastus medialis**, **vastus intermedius** (not visible), and **rectus femoris**.

When it comes to knowing the muscles of the quads, all you need to know is that there are four of them, and if you are looking to get well-defined thighs, you will want to show separation between these muscles, which is done mostly through having a low enough body fat percentage.

Quadriceps Function

The quadriceps stretch over the knee and hip joints, so they can cause movement at both locations. The quads perform two main functions:

1. Extend and straighten the leg at the knee
2. Flex (bend) the hips, such as by raising the leg to the chest
3. Whenever you need to straighten your knee, it's your quads that come into play. Imagine kicking a ball or jumping.

For example, when you perform a squat, it's your quadriceps that take most of the strain at the beginning of the effort as you are bending your knees. The farther you go down, the more you will bend at the hips and cause the glutes to take a lot of stress as well. As you straighten back up, your knees extend and your quads flex.

Quadriceps Training

To train your quads fully, you will need compound movements with a full range of motion, and most likely a single-joint leg extension as well.

Compound leg exercises will not only help you build strong, good-looking quads but will also help you develop a strong core by tightening your abdominal muscles and spinal erectors to keep your spine stable throughout the movement. The compound exercises will build the most muscles and the most strength, which can carry over to everyday life and other lifts. When you do them with a full range of motion as dictated by your body, you will also build flexibility in your hips, knees, and ankles.

To target the inside or outside muscles of the quads, you can adjust your foot placement for exercises like the squat or leg press. But research has shown that the overall development of certain areas is minimal and it is more important to create mechanical tension over the whole quad than it is to try to isolate the different muscles.

Finally, the rectus femoris, which is the large front-and-center quad muscle, stretches across your hip. This means that when your hips are bent, such as when you are squatting, they will not receive much tension. Therefore, you might want to add an isolation leg-extension exercise to your program. If you allow your hips to extend, you will nicely target your mid-quad. You can do this by moving the back pad of a standard leg-extension machine farther back so you are leaning backward more.

THE HAMSTRINGS

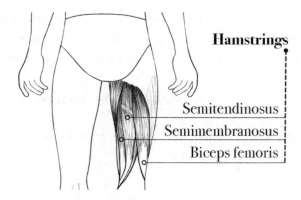

Hamstrings

Semitendinosus
Semimembranosus
Biceps femoris

PRIMARY HAMSTRING EXERCISES

· Romanian deadlift	· Leg curl	· Glute-ham raise
· Hip thrust	· Cable pull-through	· Hip extension

The hamstrings are the muscles located on the back of the thigh. They attach at the hip and below the knee.

The hamstrings are composed of the **biceps femoris**, **semitendinosus**, and **semimembranosus**.

The biceps femoris is the largest and most prominent muscle of the hamstring. On well-developed hamstrings, the biceps femoris and the semitendinosus will be the most visually present, and appear as two long muscles running side-by-side down the thigh.

Overall, the hamstrings are often trained as one single muscle, since the muscles tend to work together. There are ways to train the individual muscles of the hamstring and the upper or lower parts of the different muscles, but all you need to know to achieve well-rounded development is the location that the exercises hit, not the exact muscles.

Hamstring Function

The hamstrings have two major functions:

1. Flex (bend) the knee
2. Extend the leg at the hip in conjunction with the glutes
3. The hamstrings are involved in movements such as squatting down (though not intensely involved), bending forward to pick up a weight, and bending your knee (curling your leg).

Hamstring Training

The hamstrings are biarticulate, which means they stretch over two joints. This feature allows them to be trained through movement of the different joints they stretch across.

When one joint is not moving (static), the other joint will be able to train the muscle. However, when both joints are moving, the muscle can't create tension and pull on a specific end of the muscle. Either that, or one end is relaxing while the other is trying to pull on it. This results in poor stress or even an inability to cause movement or tension. It's like relaxing one end of a rubber band while the other is trying to stretch.

The hamstrings come into effect with almost every compound movement that involves the legs. But these exercises are highly quad- and glute-dominant, so the hamstrings receive minimal training. This is why you will need to include hamstring-specific movements.

To train the hamstrings, you'll need to perform leg-curling and hip-extension motions like the seated leg curl and the Romanian deadlift (RDL) or cable pull-through. Hip-extension exercises will help increase muscle mass due to the amount of weight that can be used. The different leg curls will isolate the different areas of your hamstrings and work the muscles' knee-flexion function.

As long as you perform at least one hip-extension exercise and one knee-flexion exercise, you will develop the backs of your thighs fully and create hamstrings that blend nicely into your glutes and quads.

THE GLUTES

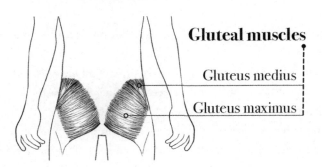

Gluteal muscles

Gluteus medius

Gluteus maximus

PRIMARY GLUTE EXERCISES		
• Squat • Romanian deadlift	• Hip thrust • Hip extension	• Lunge • Leg abduction

The glutes are very important for everyday life. They are used in almost all sports, help with other lifts, and keep you from getting hurt when you do other exercises that don't focus on the glutes.

To optimally develop your whole butt, you will need to concentrate on only two major muscles. Of course, there are muscles underneath and different muscle functions that these muscles perform, but there are only two muscles that can be seen visually.

The **gluteus maximus**, also referred to as the glutes, are the large buttock muscles. The gluteus maximus is the main muscle you should concentrate on.

The **gluteus medius** is located above the gluteus maximus and on the outer thigh/hip.

Beneath the gluteus medius is the gluteus minimus, which works in conjunction with the other muscles and can't be directly targeted.

Glute Function

The gluteus maximus is a large muscle with many different attachment locations and muscle fiber angles, so it completes or helps with a lot of different movements and functions. These are the major ones:
Straightening the hips, such as in standing up from a seated position

1. Extending the legs and kicking them back behind the body
2. Rotating the upper leg at the hip, both inward and outward, in a motion similar to the butterfly stretch
3. Abducting the leg (extending it to the side), but mainly when the hips are bent

The gluteus medius helps the gluteus maximus in some of its functions, but it is also the primary muscle used in these motions:

1. Extending the leg out to the side, mostly when the hips are straight. This is known as abduction, or movement away from the center of the body.
2. Rotating the upper leg outward and inward

Whenever there is movement at the hips, the glutes come into play.

Glute Training

Since the glutes have so many different muscle fibers that attach to many different locations, to train your glutes fully, you can include enough exercises to stress the upper and lower fibers, the hyperextension function, and the abduction function.

However, for most males, glute-specific work is not necessary or desired to give you well-rounded buttocks. You can often get away without any extra glute-specific training.

Instead, it's more beneficial to perform multi-joint exercises that require you to straighten your bent hips. The main exercises that straighten fully bent or flexed hips are the RDL, hip thrust, and squat (surprising, I know).

In all, simply doing squats and RDLs through a full range of motion, to allow for a full glute stretch and hip bend, will provide you with enough glute training to fill out your jeans and round out your physique. You can add in hip thrusts or abduction exercises as needed.

THE BICEPS

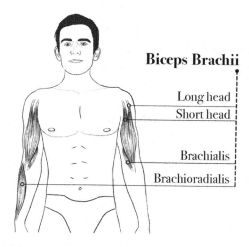

Biceps Brachii

Long head
Short head

Brachialis
Brachioradialis

PRIMARY BICEPS EXERCISES

- Single-arm curl
- EZ-bar or barbell curl

- Seated dumbbell incline curl

- Preacher curl

For males, the biceps are often among the most trained muscles. It's common for new weight lifters to spend too much time doing curls and not enough time working on other muscle groups, making the biceps look disproportionate, like Popeye's overly ballooned arms.

The biceps is a two-headed muscle more scientifically called the **biceps brachii**. The **biceps brachii** originates under the deltoid and inserts below the elbow.

The biceps brachii are the major muscles of the front of the upper arms and are responsible for a majority of the functions performed by the upper arm, but there are two other muscles that are often included when discussing the biceps. These are the **brachialis** and **brachioradialis**. The brachialis is beneath the biceps brachii and is only visible on the outer (lateral) side of the arm when you are very lean. The brachioradialis crosses from the upper arm over the elbow and onto the forearm.

Biceps Function

The biceps has two major functions:

1. To lift and curl the arm at the elbow
2. To rotate the forearm

The biceps helps with multi-joint back movements whenever the forearm gets pulled toward the upper arm, as in pulling motions. This is important to understand because it is often overlooked when determining total training volume for the biceps. In general, if you are flexing your arm with resistance, you will need to use your biceps to complete the motion.

The biceps also has the function of rotating the lower arm outward and inward. Picture your palms facing down and rotating until they're facing up, and vice versa. The brachioradialis works in conjunction with the biceps brachii to curl and flex the elbow and to rotate the lower arm, but can only rotate to a neutral position.

Biceps Training

To develop the biceps to their full potential, you do not need to train for mass, length, peak, inside and outside, upper and lower, etc., like some influencers or bodybuilders would have you believe.

The two heads of your biceps brachii, the outer (lateral) long head and the inner (medial) short head, are trained whenever you complete a pulling motion, like when training your back muscles. Most men don't realize that they don't need to do as many extra biceps isolation exercises if they focus on progression, proper volume, and technique.

To isolate the long head of your biceps even more, you can do a curl with your arm behind your back, like a cable curl with your back to the cable machine.

Curls with your arm in front of your body for isolation of the short head of the biceps, like preacher curls, can be added as desired, but this head of the muscle will already be worked with pull-ups, pull-downs, rows, upright rows, etc.

Neutral-grip elbow-flexion movements, such as hammer curls, will stress your brachioradialis maximally, along with your biceps brachii.

THE TRICEPS

Triceps Brachii

Long head
Lateral head
Medial head

PRIMARY TRICEPS EXERCISES

- Close-grip bench press
- Dip

- Skullcrusher
- Overhead triceps extension

- Triceps extension variations

When a person has truly massive arms, it is the triceps that create that effect. When flexed, the triceps looks like a horseshoe on the back of the arm.

The triceps is a three-headed muscle composed of the long, medial, and lateral heads. The triceps is larger in size than the biceps and should take up about two-thirds of the upper arm.

Scientifically called the **triceps brachii**, the triceps attaches under the deltoid and below the elbow.

Triceps Function

The triceps works in opposition to the biceps. It has one major function: to straighten the arm at the elbow.

The long head of the triceps is the primary extender of your elbow when your upper arm is raised. The medial and lateral heads of the triceps work together to straighten your arm when your elbow is close to or by your side.

Whenever you do a pushing motion or a straightening of the arm under resistance, your triceps helps. So, in movements like the bench press and shoulder press, you will also get help from your triceps—though the triceps might not get worked through a full range of motion.

Triceps Training

Since the triceps has three heads as compared to two for the biceps, the triceps needs to be trained from more angles. Still, similar to the biceps, the triceps doesn't need excessive work to be developed fully.

To isolate the medial and lateral heads of the triceps, you can add a push-down motion with your elbows close to your sides, like a single-arm extension.

You'll also need to add a triceps extension with your arm raised, like an overhead triceps extension or skullcrusher, to isolate the long head of the triceps. During compound pressing movements for other muscle groups, the long head of the triceps receives less stress than the other heads.

It's important not to train the triceps before training a bigger muscle group that will use the triceps, like the chest or shoulders.

THE ABDOMINALS

Abdominals

- External obliques
- Rectus abdominis
- Transverse abdominis

PRIMARY ABDOMINAL EXERCISES

• Reverse crunch and variations	• Crunch and variations • Plank and side plank	• Oblique twist

Strong abdominals, more commonly referred to as your abs, core, or midsection, are essential for performance in almost any sport and in daily life.

For an impressive physique, it's necessary to have well-defined abs. They are the visual center of the body and a true sign that you work hard both in the gym and with your diet.

Apart from losing any excess abdominal fat, you may also need to train your abs with some isolation work. This is where a lot of mistakes are made—a lot.

Most people don't know how the abs actually work and don't realize that there is more to abs than the standard six-pack muscles.

Visually, the abdominals are composed of the **rectus abdominis** and the **external obliques**.

The **rectus abdominis** is the muscle that forms the sought-after six-pack. It is a long muscle that starts in the pubis (the bone at the bottom of the pelvis) and ends in the cartilage of the ribs.

The **external obliques** are located on the sides of the torso. They are attached to the pelvis and ribs.

Under the external abdominal muscles are the **transverse abdominis** and the internal obliques. The transverse abdominis is an important muscle to train, but the internal obliques are less important.

The transverse abdominis attaches between the pelvis and ribs and extends around your midsection.

Abdominal Function

The rectus abdominis has two functions:

1. To flex the spinal column and draw the sternum toward the pelvis in a crunching motion
2. To tilt the pelvis toward the sternum in a reverse crunching motion

The obliques:

1. Flex and rotate the spinal column.
2. Flex the spine to the side in a crunching motion.

The main function of the transverse abdominis is spinal stabilization through flexing and tightening the core.

When the abdominal muscles contract, they pull the rib cage and the pelvis toward each other in a crunching motion. The role of the abs is simply to crunch the rib cage and pelvis together in a short movement. That is it.

So, any movement that does not require either the pelvis to crunch to the rib cage or the rib cage to crunch to the pelvis is not a primary ab exercise. For example, when a person does a sit-up, the main movement is in the hips. The primary muscles being used are not the abs but the iliopsoas muscles—the hip flexors.

Abdominal Training

The abdominal muscles work not only to crunch the rib cage to the pelvis but also to stabilize and rotate the spinal column.

To prevent creating a blocky midsection that diminishes your V taper, you want to keep your core lean and tight by avoiding excessive abdominal training. Instead, concentrate on the spinal stabilization function of your transverse abdominis by lifting heavy weights that load your spinal column. These could be exercises like squats, deadlifts, and standing shoulder presses. By tightening and flexing your core as you complete these exercises, you will maintain proper form, protect your spinal column, and develop a strong midsection that remains lean and flat. This is similar to doing abdominal planks but with better results and carryover to other lifts.

When it comes to abdominal-specific exercises, you need to train both the front and the sides of your torso. For training your visible abs properly, variations of crunches and twists will isolate different areas of your midsection for great overall development.

To train your upper abs best, you should do any variation of the common crunch. To train your lower abs, you can do a reverse crunch variation, in which you curl your hips up instead of your chest.

When it comes to the sides of your torso, perform oblique twists, side planks, or side crunches with little to no weight.

THE CALVES

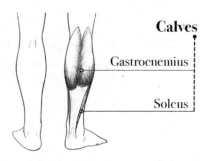

• Standing calf raise	• Seated calf raise

Calves are often considered the most difficult muscle group to develop. For proper proportion, the calves should be about the same size as the biceps, but often the calves are neglected or not trained enough to develop size.

While calf training can help create muscular and fit lower legs, the skinniness of your ankles will be determined by your genetic joint size and your body fat level, since the ankle area is bone, not muscle. Still, your calves need to be trained and developed.

The calves are composed of two muscles: the **soleus** and the **gastrocnemius**.

The **soleus** is the longer and deeper of the two calf muscles. The **gastrocnemius** is two-headed and originates from the femur. The gastrocnemius is the part of the calf that looks like an upside-down heart and grows the most.

Calf Function

The calves are used to flex and extend the foot. The gastrocnemius extends the foot when the knee is straight. Whenever you walk, run, or jump, your calves come into action to help you push off the ground and extend your feet to move yourself.

When the knee is bent, the gastrocnemius cannot function due to relaxation at both ends of its muscle attachment. This is where the soleus comes into play and takes over the movement.

Calf Training

Calf training tends to be highly individualized. You will need to determine what works best for your body and train accordingly.

Your calves are used to working whenever you run and walk, so they tend to have great endurance. Therefore, you need to put your calves under a lot of stress in order to overload them.

The main mass-building exercise for calves is the standing calf raise. Any calf exercise in which the leg is straight will work the more visible gastrocnemius.

Seated calf raises or any bent-knee exercise will isolate the longer soleus.

THE FOREARMS

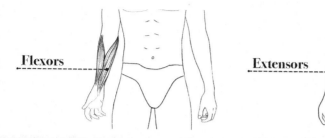

PRIMARY FOREARM EXERCISES

· Pulling exercises	· Wrist curl

The forearm muscles make up the lower part of the arm. They are involved in nearly every exercise for the upper body. The **forearm** comprises a variety of muscles on the outside and inside of the lower arm.

Forearm Function

The forearm is composed of flexor and extensor muscles. The forearm has two functions:

1. The flexor muscles curl the palm down and forward.
2. The extensor muscles curl the knuckles back and up.

The forearms help with almost every upper-body exercise by either helping grip the equipment or being a part of the pushing and pulling actions.

Forearm Training

Since the forearms are involved in nearly every upper-body exercise, they often get trained through having to grip the weight.

If you notice that a lack of grip strength is holding you back during some exercises, you should include more forearm training with an emphasis on grip strength.

In general, you can get away with not doing any extra forearm work. Most of the time, if you train your forearms too much and do more isolation work, they will get tired or cause wrist problems. This will make it hard for you to train other muscles.

PART IV

THE ROUTINE

SECRET 7

–

SETTING THE STAGE FOR CONTINUOUS IMPROVEMENTS

CHAPTER 21

LAYING THE GROUNDWORK
FOR ACCELERATED RESULTS

It's important to remember that continued progress is vital when it comes to strength training and dieting. No one wants to work hard only to fail to see any results from their hard work, and you don't want to let any initial momentum go to waste by not committing to your program.

One of the most challenging parts of any new journey is consistency. As with any goal you are trying to achieve, you need to stay on track and work every day, every week, every month, and so on. It takes a lot of dedication and persistence to achieve your goals, and the same goes for fitness goals.

But this is also the most rewarding part of strength training; there is no feeling quite like noticing your body changing and morphing into your ideal body.

You will begin to feel your strength, fitness, endurance, and energy increase. In addition, working out releases endorphins—nervous-system hormones that reduce your perception of pain and set off positive feelings throughout your body.

Lifting weights and eating a healthy, nutritious diet also improves your overall well-being and can reduce your risk of diabetes, fight osteoporosis, limit the effects of depression, drastically increase your heart health, and much more.

Even if the changes are small and incremental, they will inspire you to carry on when you notice them.

To ensure that you are on track with your goals and making continued progress every week, you will need to keep up-to-date with your progress and be on top of your preparation. This may seem like an annoying thing to do at first, but it will very quickly become second nature, and the more progress you see, the more you will want to record it and keep preparing.

It essentially feels like you are studying yourself; you need to take notes on your exercises, weight, meals, what feels good, what needs work, and how you can improve.

The time and energy you invest in yourself and your growth are partly why this journey is so rewarding; it's a testament to your dedication, hard work, and resilience.

To progress effectively from week to week, you will need to make certain things part of your daily and weekly routine.

CHAPTER 22

THE POWER OF ROUTINE

Building an impressive physique is not the same as simply being fit. Creating the body you want takes dedication, hard work, adherence over the long term, programming, and concentration in both the weight room and the kitchen.

As we discussed at the beginning of the book, strength training is much different from exercising, and flexible dieting is not the same as healthy eating. Both strength training and flexible dieting require more effort, focus, and attention but reap far greater rewards.

Having to also concentrate on what you're doing throughout the rest of your day and how each little action might affect your training and dieting outcomes would require far too much mental energy and create excessive stress. But if you can put your day on autopilot, you can focus more on making sure you're progressing properly in your training program and that you're getting the right amounts of calories, macronutrients, and food.

Even more importantly, you will be able to reduce your stress, free up mental space for other important things, make your life more efficient, and give yourself more available time to do what you enjoy while also being mentally present for it.

To get compounding results from your strength-training and nutrition programs, you need to stay consistent. Developing muscle and strength while leaning out takes months, even years, and can be achieved only with consistent effort, consistent improvement, and sustained work toward a specific goal.

Consistency is key in building an aesthetic body, and your lifestyle, routine, and ability to maintain a stable biorhythm are the keys to consistency.

CONSISTENT LIFESTYLE FACTORS

To make progress, you need to improve your workouts and diet, but your lifestyle also needs to complement your goals if you're to gain muscle and lose fat. In addition, sufficient recovery time between training sessions for the same muscles is essential.

Fortunately, adequate recovery has been built into the workout plans provided for you in this book, but if you are changing the workouts or moving on to a more intense plan, make sure you're still getting enough recovery time.

Controlling stress is another important lifestyle factor. Stress is related to an uptick in levels of the hormone cortisol, and a long-term increase in cortisol can wreak havoc on your whole hormonal system. High and sustained stress can ramp up fat gain and undermine strength gains.

Sleep deprivation is even worse for you than chronic stress. Lack of sleep can cause all sorts of health problems and reduce your performance in and out of the gym. Making sure you get enough sleep each night is the first step, so work that into your schedule.

The second thing is to improve the quality of your sleep. Scheduling 8 hours of sleep a night is good on paper, but if you're not getting enough deep sleep and rapid eye movement (REM) sleep, you can still be sleep deprived.

STRESS VERSUS ROUTINE

When it comes to training and dieting to develop your physique, psychological stress has been shown to cause:[1,2]

- Increased appetite.

- Cravings for comfort foods.

- Poor carb tolerance and impaired nutrient partitioning.

- Far lower strength development.

- Far slower recovery after exercise.

- Reduced muscle growth.

- Increased risk of injury.

Training has a dual role when it comes to stress. On the one hand, it reduces psychological (mental) stress, and on the other, it causes physiological (body) stress.

When you do light exercise, endorphins are released, which can help you feel less stressed. But intense exercise can add even more stress. Though these are two different forms of stress, they both affect your recovery.

So, to get the best results possible, you need to keep your stress levels low. Of course, this may seem easier said than done, especially if you have a lot going on in your professional and personal life.

The first and most important thing you should do is work to lower your stress levels by creating a routine, improving your health through diet and exercise, getting better sleep, and using other stress-reducing strategies.

Although it's sometimes thought to put you in a rut, creating an easy-to-follow, mindless "rut"-ine will reduce decision fatigue and stress, allowing you to concentrate on more important things in your life. Look to form a routine with your training schedule, meal composition and prep, meal timing, sleep, and more.

Most of the time, the best way to deal with stress is to have a solid routine that keeps your life in balance. The best routines begin with slowly forming or changing habits, which are your regular tendencies or practices.

Start with improving your sleep by making your nighttime and morning habits more conducive to sleeping and waking up. Make a habit of heading to bed at the same time every night and getting enough sleep every night.

Next, stabilize your body's biorhythm and slowly work to maintain your daily eating and training habits.

All these habits should become a routine that can help you cool down your chronic stress levels, boost your recovery, and improve your muscle-building, fat-loss, and strength-training progression.

IMPROVE SLEEP ROUTINE

As you probably know at this point in your life, sleep is vital for your health and longevity. Yet many people don't realize just how crucial sleep is to their physique goals. It's often overlooked as something you just do every night, but you can really hamper your progress by undersleeping.

When it comes to building a great body, here are just some of the proven adverse effects of sleep deprivation:

- Poor use of protein and other nutrients[3]

- Decreased testosterone production[4]

- Higher stress levels[5]

- Increased resistance to insulin[6]

- Slower metabolism[7]

- Increased appetite and less self-control[8]

- Impaired cognitive functioning[9]

- Decreased well-being[10]

Without a proper bedtime, sleep, and early morning routine, which helps you create a stable circadian rhythm, consistently getting enough deep sleep can be difficult. And when I say enough, I mean enough—the ideal recommended number of hours, not just the amount you can survive on. The fact that you can function on 5 to 6 hours of sleep a night does not mean that it is healthy. You may have gotten used to it, but that doesn't mean your body recovers faster. Your muscles and cognitive function may still be hindered, and you won't even know it because you have "gotten used to it."

The typical recommendation for sleep is 7 to 8 hours per night—but this is for sedentary individuals. As a hard strength trainer, you'll probably require more. On the other hand, hard training improves sleep quality.

So, you should shoot for 8 to 9 hours of sleep nightly to reap the full benefits of improved sleep and meet your need for more recovery time.

If you struggle with getting enough sleep, you should first maintain a regular sleeping, eating, and training schedule.

To begin with, reduce your caffeine intake, especially near bedtime. And before bed:

- Limit bright light and blue light.

- Limit fluid intake.

- Avoid foods that interfere with your sleep.

- Possibly take a warm bath or shower.

Lower your bedroom temperature at night and improve your sleeping atmosphere with sound-proofing or white noise, blackout shades, and a more comfortable bed.

Upon waking, aim for daily sunlight exposure, even if it's from a light lamp, as close to waking up as possible.

All these measures will help improve your sleep routine, rein in your stress levels, and create a stable circadian rhythm.

Maintaining a Stable Biorhythm

Your internal clock regulates a 24-hour cycle of biological activity known as your circadian rhythm, or biorhythm. Your circadian rhythm affects a wide range of systems, including your sleep-wake cycle.

In general, your body's biorhythm will affect every system in your body, because your body likes to stay in homeostasis. One of the best ways for your body to maintain homeostasis is to be prepared for what's coming next. This is what routines and habits are based on. They take the thinking and stress out of everyday tasks and let your body use its internal clock to put your life on autopilot.

In fact, even when sleep isn't optimized, a stable biorhythm characterized by regular mealtimes, morning caffeine use with exposure to light, and an exercise routine can enhance cognitive function, physical performance, and general well-being.[11]

So, apart from your sleep schedule, having a diet-and-nutrition routine can have huge effects on your muscle and strength gains and your body's ability to lose fat without even adjusting each program variable.

Maintain a Regular Training Schedule

The people who struggle the most with sticking with a training program are the people who fit their training into their schedule as an afterthought. Everything else takes priority, but if they have an extra hour, they will make it to the gym.

These same people are the ones who desire the mental and physical health benefits that come from maintaining a consistent training routine but aren't willing to make slight adjustments to make their lives easier. But again, a routine serves to make your life efficient and more manageable, not to keep you from social events, family time, relaxation at home, etc.

So, you need to not just make training a priority, but make it a part of your lifestyle such that, if missed, it will throw off the rest of your routine.

For this reason, in general, I always recommend that the number of days you train each week should be the total number of days you are willing and able to go to the gym or train. If you are willing and able to go to the gym six times a week, you should strength train six days a week.

Also, try to go to the gym at the same time every workout day, at an hour that suits your body's circadian rhythm and around which you can time your meals appropriately. This will help you form a routine, get you exercising as many days as possible, help with mental health, and give you the ability to spread out your training volume, which can make your training sessions shorter, to carve out more time for "fun" activities.

Maintain Regular Eating Times

Sticking with a consistent meal pattern is highly beneficial for regulating your appetite, preventing unplanned snacking, improving fat loss, and improving your health.[12,13,14]

In fact, whether you eat breakfast or skip it, it doesn't affect your physique as long as you do it consistently and maintain a meal pattern throughout the rest of your day.[15]

So, eat your meals at fixed times, and once you've determined your meal timing, stick to it. Don't snack when you don't have snack time on your schedule.

If you are consistent and let it turn into a habit, you will realize that you feel hungry only at the times you are accustomed to eating. That's because hunger becomes a function of habit. If you always snack at 3:00 p.m., your internal clock will release ghrelin, the "hunger hormone," to tell you that it's 3:00 p.m. and it's time to eat.

WEEKLY ROUTINES

The previous topics were related to your daily life. But there are specific tasks that might take place only once, maybe twice a week. These weekly tasks, which should become a routine in themselves, provide the guidelines for many daily tasks. The weekly tasks take stock of the previous week, analyze it, and make adjustments for the upcoming week.

By implementing daily routines and following them up with weekly routines to determine what's working and what's not and to prepare for the next week, your life will run even smoother. You'll keep improving your routine, physique, and well-being without much effort.

We'll discuss these in separate chapters, but here is what you should be doing each week:

- Tracking and measuring your progress, routine, well-being, and current body composition

- Adjusting your meal plan based on the results you're getting physically and mentally

- Prepping meals in advance as needed and preferred for staying organized and preventing unnecessary stress

- Adjusting your strength-training program based on results and preparation for the coming week

CHAPTER 23

THE CORRECT WAYS TO TRACK AND MEASURE BODY CHANGES

The switch from simply exercising and lifting weights to legitimately training requires programming. So, whether you are looking to train for pure strength, to pack on muscle mass, or to sculpt an aesthetic physique, you need to create a program that can get you there.

This demands knowing where you are currently, having a clear vision of your end goal, understanding what you need to adjust to get your current body to your end goal, creating a training and nutrition program to get you there, and consistently measuring and tracking to determine whether you're doing everything correctly or if you might need to make adjustments to your program.

By taking consistent measurements and tracking them over time, you'll be able to understand if what you're doing is working or if you might need to pivot to get back on track.

In this chapter, we'll go over the various things you should measure and track and how to do it correctly and efficiently. This will help you implement the strength-training and nutrition variables in the upcoming sections.

When you understand what you should be mindful of each week and how to measure changes in your body, you'll understand what you might need to fix or slightly tweak in your strength-training program and meal plan for better results.

Don't worry—you don't need excessive measuring methods or have to track every little pound on the scale and the barbell. But you do need a measuring routine that helps you track your progress toward your goal.

That last part is important. Tracking progress isn't just a tool for elite lifters or those who dedicate their lives to the pursuit of creating a statuesque body. Instead, it's a tool that helps you maintain your focus on why you started this journey in the first place and puts into perspective just how far you have come.

If you set up a routine for measuring and keeping track of your progress and stick to it, you are more likely to make strength training and eating healthy a way of life instead of a chore or a necessary evil.

YOUR TWO METHODS FOR MEASURING PROGRESS

You will use both internal and external measuring methods for tracking your progress.

You'll measure improvements based on feelings, both psychological and physical. This feedback from internal sources takes a subjective approach.

Since emotions and feelings aren't always accurate and can lead you astray, you'll also use measurable and quantifiable methods to help you figure out how your body composition has changed. This feedback from external sources requires a completely analytical approach.

Together, they will provide a complete representation of where you are, what's improved, what hasn't, and what needs to change moving forward.

Then, in upcoming chapters, we'll go over how to adjust your programs to keep getting results or improve the results you are seeing.

Determine which method will work for you and stay consistent with it every single week. Then, if at any time you are unable to stick to the tracking and measuring, switch to an easier method or take a break for as long as you need to.

Let's start by determining your starting point so you always have something to compare to and see just how far you have actually come. Then we'll look at how to measure and track changes from there.

Record Your Starting Physique

A very beneficial way to ensure that you stay on track and don't get disheartened when times might seem tough (or when you don't feel like dieting or training) is to take photos of yourself at the very beginning of your journey.

That way, as you progress, you can look back at how far you've come and realize that the hard work has been worth it. You can see that you are truly getting results, even if you don't feel you have made much progress some days or weeks.

You may not notice the tiny changes in your body because you're used to looking at it every day, so referring back to your "before" photos is a necessary reminder that you are changing your body composition.

You should take the pictures in the morning, before eating and after using the bathroom. The best lighting comes from natural light or consistent artificial light, as long as it is always the same. This is because different types of lighting can significantly change how you look.

Take photos straight on, from the side, and from the back. Wear shorts or underwear so you can see your whole body. Take pictures of yourself in as relaxed a state as possible; these are for your own private reference, so you need to be honest with yourself.

You may also take photos while flexed to see muscle development and any other changes that start to show. Just be sure to compare the correct pictures for an accurate reading.

Similarly, you should determine your initial body weight. Weigh yourself and record it in your phone, workout journal, app, or wherever you prefer. The best time to weigh yourself is the same as for taking photos—in the morning, before eating and after using the bathroom.

How to Measure Using Internal Feedback

Determining how well your diet and training programs are working can be as simple as tracking how you're feeling from day to day and week to week. Although this is highly subjective, the benefits of feeling better can't be understated, especially since this maintains simplicity and reduces the mental stress that other measuring methods can cause.

If you are just starting out with measuring your body changes and tracking them weekly, or you simply aren't interested in anything besides working out and eating better, then you should use internal feedback to make any program adjustments.

The major things to pay attention to, as you can use them to adjust your nutrition and training programs, are:

- Hunger and diet enjoyability.

- Performance in the gym.

- Health and well-being.

If you are always hungry or your current meal plan is a struggle to stick to, you will most likely need to adjust your diet to be more sustainable. This can also include making changes in your ability to measure and track your food intake and building more confidence in your ability to diet. Be sure to jot down any struggles you're having with your current meal plan wherever you are tracking your progress.

Next, you should track how well you're performing in the gym from week to week and sometimes even session to session.

The improvements you're looking for include that you feel stronger; you're able to breathe easier while working out; you're recovering faster between sets; you're not feeling as tired during a workout or as sore afterward; your technique has improved; you're more coordinated; and you're becoming more flexible and increasing your range of motion.

Finally, and most importantly, track your health and well-being. Strength training and maintaining a quality diet should almost always improve your overall health and well-being. If you feel this is not the case, you should make a huge adjustment in one program or both.

Tracking Methods for Measuring Body Composition

Improving based on feel and internal feedback can't be underestimated. Both can be very important markers for long-term transformation.

However, these don't provide a completely accurate picture of how your body composition is changing. You need to be able to accurately and objectively track your changes in strength, muscle mass, and body fat.

So, using other measurement methods to corroborate your results is important. But these methods shouldn't be difficult to put into practice. Instead, they should be quick and easily repeatable, with little possibility of being misleading.

Very few progress-measuring methods fit these requirements, so you will use photos and body-weight measurements. Both are simple, fast, and repeatable.

These will be combined with your strength progression, which is done by measuring your increases in training weights each training session. We'll discuss this when we implement the training variables in the next section.

You should look for three things when comparing your strength, body weight, and physique photos. First, your strength is increasing on primary lifts.

The best way to measure progress is in the gym, under the bar. If you're getting stronger week to week and month to month, you're improving. In theory, if you can consistently improve your strength on primary lifts, then you are most likely building muscle. If not, you probably need to adjust your diet and/or training program.

Second, your body weight is moving in the direction you desire (more than likely decreasing slowly). The change in body weight, as measured by a digital bathroom scale, is a good way to tell if you are losing or gaining fat. You should use this measurement mainly to adjust your meal plan, calorie intake, and protein intake.

But be aware, body weight can be very misleading. Are you losing fat, muscle, water, or a combination? Or is your body losing fat but gaining muscle, so the scale is hardly budging?

For this reason, you'll also take weekly physique photos. So, the third thing you should look for is whether you appear leaner and more muscular in your photos.

Pictures can be highly inaccurate and misinterpreted, but when combined with the other two measuring methods, weekly photos can help you track changes in your muscle mass and body fat.

All three of these markers are basic signs of positive body recomposition. However, if you fail one or more of these, you might need to adopt more accurate measuring methods, allow more time for adaptations and adjustments, or alter your training and diet.

Your Measuring and Tracking Routine

To implement proper measuring and tracking, you should have a journal, notepad, workout app, food tracking app, or any other medium that allows you to quickly and easily mark down how you're feeling, your body weight, your weights for training, and your food intake.

Here is what you should keep track of and use to create a routine:

- Note internal cues each day or as often as needed.

- Track your food intake (discussed in the meal-plan creation section).

- Track your training weights (discussed in the strength-training implementation section).

- Weigh yourself at least once weekly.

- Take physique photos once weekly or every other week.

When weighing yourself and taking photos, you will need to keep taking the same measurements every week on the same day at the same time. Set an alarm on measurement day—I would suggest Sunday morning—and take 5 to 10 minutes to weigh yourself and take progress photos. Then record your weight in your notepad or note-taking app.

When you weigh yourself, keep your specific weight-change goals in mind so you can adjust your program as your weight changes, if necessary.

Weighing yourself at the same time and on the same day each week, before eating and after using the bathroom, is important for consistency.

Next, take weekly progress photos under the same lighting and in the same state as your initial photos. You won't be able to track your progress accurately if you aren't keeping every factor within your control the same each measuring time.

The best thing to do is to put all these photos in a specific folder so they're easy to find in your camera roll.

You may not see changes over a single week, but if you are consistent with your program, routine, and strength progression, you will be able to observe noticeable changes when you compare photos multiple weeks apart.

PART V

THE APPLICATION

SECRET 8

-

DESIGNING A TRAINING PROGRAM FOR BUILDING AN AMAZING BODY

CHAPTER 24

HOW TO IMPLEMENT THE TRAINING PROGRAM VARIABLES

So far, we've covered everything you need to know to build muscles through strength training. This section is where we apply all the knowledge and training variables.

In this chapter, we'll talk about the basic steps for putting volume, intensity, and frequency into action to create a training program. By starting with only the correct number of weekly sets per muscle (volume), reps and resistance (intensity), and number of days you train a muscle (frequency), you will be able to put all your focus into forming a solid foundation of muscle, strength, and neuromuscular coordination through perfecting the most important variables first.

In order to apply these variables correctly and get maximal results, the name of the game is consistency—consistency in following your schedule, maintaining your effort level, doing the exercises right, getting more confident in your training, and growing stronger with each workout.

This might sound extremely easy, especially if you have been working out for a while now, but a lack of respect for the basics and a failure to form a proper foundation are the reasons a lot of men fail to get results. In fact, the people who often need this chapter the most are the men who have been lifting weights for a while now but have seen very little success.

Nobody cares how long you've been going to the gym or how many books you've read. If you don't have the muscles and strength to prove it, then there is a major disconnect in how you are implementing the information you've read in all those books.

Alternatively, you might just want to make sure you have the most important variables correct, but you don't care about taking that next step and dialing in your program even more. This is often the case for the average gym-goer who wants to be healthy and fit but is willing to sacrifice results for simplicity.

Some men might get all the results they want without needing to add more complexity and implement more complex training variables. The other men will simply use this as a stepping stone toward an amazing body and a long training career.

In the chapters after this, we will get into the *Physique Secrets* programs, recommended exercises, and how to adjust your program to better fit your situation.

First, let's lay out the basic steps for applying the training program variables. Most of the logical thinking has been done for you; all you need to understand is how everything fits together so you can adjust it as needed.

STEP #0: ESTABLISH A DESTINATION

Before you begin, you need to set a realistic end goal and determine what improvements you want or need to make. Strength training and working to build an amazing body is a bit different from other activities in that specific goals are limited by your genetic capabilities.

Packing on 20 pounds of muscle might be easy for a man who has never worked out and is 6'4" with a large skeletal frame and big joints. But a 5'7" man with small joints who is an intermediate-level trainee might be lucky to gain 10 pounds of muscle over the course of a year.

Instead of setting an unrealistic end goal, determine which of your muscles to prioritize for strength and growth based on your preferences, which muscle groups you might be lacking in compared to others, and which exercises you want to get stronger in compared to others.

STEP #1: DETERMINE HOW OFTEN YOU'LL TRAIN

The number of days you train per week should be simple to determine because it will correspond to your regular schedule.

This is something we talked about in the section on making a routine, but try to train as many days as you can, even if you have to cut some sessions short because of time.

STEP #2: DETERMINE TRAINING FREQUENCY PER MUSCLE

In order to spread out your sets and exercises, you should start by establishing how many times a week you'll train each muscle. This will allow you to match your training frequency, sets, exercises, and rest days to the training schedule you determined in step 1.

You should train each muscle at least twice a week, with at most three or four days between training sessions for that muscle.

It's important to remember that the recommended training frequency for each muscle group is more of a minimum than an ideal. So, you can train some muscles slightly more frequently than others (as long as you do the correct number of sets).

STEP #3: DETERMINE THE OPTIMAL NUMBER OF SETS PER MUSCLE

In general, you want to be using the maximum number of sets that your body and muscles can handle while still being able to recover and progress in strength and size.

However, it's important to understand that this is over the long term. You might feel great in one training session and think that your body can handle more sets that day, but drastically increasing your total number of sets will affect your future training sessions and progress. Instead, on your above-average days, work to complete more repetitions instead of more sets.

If you are just starting strength training or are relatively new to it, begin with 12 sets per muscle per week for your upper body and 9 to 12 sets for your lower body.

If you've been training consistently for three to six months and have solid technique, do 14 sets for your upper body and 12 to 14 for your lower body each week.

If you've been consistently training hard for six months or longer, do 16 sets weekly for upper-body muscles and 14 to 16 for lower-body muscles.

STEP #4: SPLIT MUSCLE GROUPS ACROSS TRAINING DAYS

In step 0 you determined where you wanted or needed to improve and which exercises you wanted or needed to get stronger in. You also know how often you'll be training and how frequently you'll train each muscle group.

Selecting exercises is difficult, since there are thousands of options to choose from. So, for right now, I highly suggest simply determining how you would like to split the different muscle groups. Then choose from the exercises that use those muscle groups, and concentrate only on hitting the correct volume and intensity for that muscle group.

The most common method is to group muscle groups that either have opposing functions, like pushing and pulling (such as the back and chest or the biceps and triceps), or have similar functions, like the pressing movements performed by the chest, shoulders, and triceps, or the pulling movements performed by the back and biceps.

Once you've determined your muscle-group split, simply spread everything out across your training days. To match your training frequency, I would suggest making one training session and doing it twice a week.

Put priority exercises first in your program, followed by compound exercises that train large muscle groups, then isolation exercises that train large muscle groups, compound exercises that train smaller muscle groups, and finally isolation exercises that train smaller muscle groups.

STEP #5: SPLIT SETS ACROSS TRAINING DAYS AND EXERCISES

Take your weekly number of sets and spread them across your exercises based on the muscles the exercise trains and how frequently you train each muscle.

If you have a training frequency of two times per week, simply split your total sets in half and place half the sets on one day and the other half on the other day. If you're training each muscle three times a week, split the total sets into thirds.

For example, if you are doing shoulders Mondays and Thursdays and have 16 total sets per week for shoulders, do 8 sets on Monday and 8 sets on Thursday.

You should do 3 or 4 sets per exercise on average to ensure that you're doing enough volume for muscle development. You can drop to 2 sets for less important exercises or go up to 5 sets to reach a specific set number.

STEP #6: DETERMINE REPETITION MINIMUMS AND TRAINING SESSION WEIGHT FOR EACH EXERCISE

In an upcoming chapter, we will add in microloading and measuring your progress, but to continue to prioritize simplicity, strength development, and consistency, you will only need to determine the lowest number of target reps for each exercise or type of exercise, e.g., compound or isolation.

The target for compound exercises will be 6 to 8 repetitions. If you are new to strength training or are relatively new to lifting heavy, start with 8 reps. Over a few months, work down to 6 reps as a target.

For isolation exercises, assign 12 to 15 reps. Start with lighter weight and higher reps, then work down from 15 to 12 reps over time.

At this stage, you don't need to write down the reps for each exercise, since you will most likely be rotating exercises and training weights.

Try to use a weight that gets you as close to that target as possible. There will be times when you might use too light a weight. When that happens, instead of stopping at your recommended number of reps, you should keep going until you are close to technical failure—this is why your target is deemed a minimum rep number.

Determining an exercise's training weight might seem daunting, but it shouldn't be. First, start with a light weight, about half the weight you think you can manage, to warm up. Do about the same number of reps you have assigned in your program while concentrating on your technique and using a steady tempo.

Next, increase the weight by 10%–20% and perform another warm-up set. Slowly increase the weight each set until you reach a heavy enough weight that you are within 2 reps of technical failure (the point when your technique fails) when you finish your minimum target reps.

This will be your working weight for this training session. Count that most recent set as set number 1 for your training session, but don't count any of your other warm-up sets.

If you increase the weight by too much at a time to the point where you can't complete your required number of reps, use a weight that is in between what you used for that failed set and your previous set. There's no need to test this new weight; just begin your working sets.

The very beginning may be a process of trial and error, but as you progress in your program by slowly adding weight to the bar each training session, any slight miscalculations will dissipate.

STEP #7: GRADUALLY MOVE FROM CONSISTENCY TO PROGRESSION

Staying consistent with your training schedule and consistently putting in the effort to get the most out of your workouts can help you develop a solid foundation of muscle, strength, lifting coordination, and strength-training awareness.

However, this is still just a foundation and can only take you so far in your fitness and nutrition journey. Eventually, you should transition from simply concentrating on staying consistent to concentrating on how to progress for continual improvement. Consistency is great for turning basic fitness into a lifestyle, but if you don't switch from trying to consistently go to the gym and work hard to consistently and strategically progressing in strength and building more muscles, you'll hit an early plateau.

Also, having a vision and goal to work toward can help you stay on track and keep working hard every single day. Basically, it drives you to keep going and keep improving yourself.

Most people exercise because they feel obligated to, which is also why most people quit relatively quickly. The people who keep going are the ones who want to improve themselves every single day, no matter how incrementally. They know they will stay consistent, but now they're working toward daily incremental progression.

If you have hit a plateau or you're advanced enough to track your weights, you have a quality lifestyle so you can consistently improve, you have good technique and a feel for the movement patterns, and you understand how to make weight and rep adjustments, then you should work on implementing progressive overload and exercise specificity, which we will discuss in upcoming chapters.

◇◇◇

The importance of hitting the correct set volume, rep and weight intensity, and muscle training frequency cannot be overstated. After all, they are the three most important strength-training variables and will provide a huge percentage of your results when done correctly.

However, I understand that creating your own program can be difficult, so I took the liberty of creating one for you based on my many years of experience.

The *Physique Secrets* programs are based on everything we've talked about in the book, and they've helped a lot of men pack on muscle mass in all the most-requested places.

Once you're ready, move to the next chapter and get into the *Physique Secrets* training programs!

CHAPTER 25

PHYSIQUE SECRETS STRENGTH-TRAINING PROGRAMS

Finally, it's time to get into the weight room and start pumping iron! This is where the rubber meets the road and everything we've talked about with regard to strength training gets put into action.

I have combined the top research studies, years of knowledge, and real-world experience to create programs that are optimal for men with varying levels of experience, equipment, and time. These programs slowly build upon each other to help you progress correctly. They are designed to provide the exact amount of stress your body needs at each level.

I know that each person might not be able to go to the gym or train six days a week due to busy schedules, family commitments, or simply not wanting to, so I included three-day, four-day, five-day, and six-day programs.

Nevertheless, I strongly advise you to train six days a week, because it helps you establish a routine, spreads out the sets and frequency for training each muscle group, and allows you to burn more calories during the week.

The first program—phase 1—is for novices and trainees who are just starting to lift heavy for the first time.

Stick to the phase 1 program for about one to three months, then decide how you want to progress. You can either lower the reps to 6 and 12 reps for compound and isolation exercises, respectively, and increase the weights, or stay at the same reps and add a few more sets for each muscle group.

Adjust only one variable at a time, never both at the same time.

The outline of the programs will be two upper-body days, separated as "push" and "pull" days, and one lower-body day, which you will repeat for a total of six training days. I have done all of the sets-per-muscle-group-per-week calculations for you and spread out the exercises to allow for optimal training intensity.

After three to six months, you should increase your sets to the upper end of the recommended number, as discussed in the section on training variables, and then move on to the phase 2 programs.

In both phases 1 and 2, each training session starts with one or two of the five main exercises. This allows you to put more effort and strength into these key mass-building moves.

Your upper-body training days rotate between prioritizing different key exercises or variations of the key exercises. You will have a chest-dominant day, a shoulder-dominant day, an outer-lat-dominant day, and an inner-lat-dominant day. This will help you keep making steady progress on the main exercises while maintaining an even and proportionate physique. Rotating your starting exercises helps you avoid developing one muscle more than others and creating lagging or overdeveloped muscles.

The lower-body training days start with calf raises. A lot of men neglect their calves because they save calf training until the very end of their workout, when their motivation has faded, meaning they are likely to either skip working their calves or simply not train them as hard as they should.

After calves, the lower-body days rotate between squats and RDLs. This allows you to prioritize quads in one session and hamstrings in the other to keep your legs balanced and proportionate.

If you give each of the main exercises as much of your effort as possible and keep progressing in strength on those exercises, you will build a lot of muscle quickly, in the perfect locations.

So, it's important that you are mentally fresh and prepared to train hard, at least on these exercises. To do this, you need to have a good attitude and do a quality warm-up that isn't too strenuous. You should also know what weight and number of reps to aim for based on your progression from the last training session.

It's also important to ensure that you have long rest periods between the main exercises. The rest for the isolation exercises isn't that important, so if you are limited on time, you can reduce it after you've completed the main exercises.

Let's get into the training programs! Here they are:

PHASE 1 PROGRAMS

Phase 1: The 6-Day Program

DAY 1: PUSH—CHEST DOMINANT

Exercise	Reps	Sets
Flat bench press	6–8	3
Dumbbell shoulder press	6–8	3
Dumbbell incline bench press	6–8	3
Lateral raise	12–15	3
Overhead triceps extension	12–15	3

DAY 2: PULL—OUTER LAT DOMINANT

Exercise	Reps	Sets
Wide-grip pull-down/pull-up	6–8	3
Reverse fly or face pull	12–15	3
Straight-arm lat pull-down	12–15	3
Wide-grip shrug	12–15	3
Biceps curl	12–15	3

DAY 3: LOWER BODY—QUAD DOMINANT

Exercise	Reps	Sets
Standing calf raise	12–15	4
Squat	6–8	3
Romanian deadlift	6–8	3
Single-leg extension	12–15	3
Lying leg curl	12–15	3

DAY 4: PUSH—SHOULDER DOMINANT

Exercise	Reps	Sets
Dumbbell shoulder press	6–8	3
Flat bench press	6–8	3
Lateral raise	12–15	3
Incline fly	12–15	3
Overhead triceps extension	12–15	3

DAY 5: PULL—INNER LAT DOMINANT

Exercise	Reps	Sets
Reverse/neutral-grip pull-up/pull-down	6–8	3
Upright row	12–15	3
Wide-grip pull-down/pull-up	6–8	3
Reverse fly or face pull	12–15	3
Hammer curl	12–15	3

DAY 6: LOWER BODY—HAMSTRING DOMINANT

Exercise	Reps	Sets
Standing calf raise	12–15	5
Romanian deadlift	6–8	3
Squat	6–8	3
Seated leg curl	12–15	3
Single-leg extension	12–15	3

Phase 1: The 5-Day Program

DAY 1: PUSH		
Exercise	Reps	Sets
Flat bench press	6-8	3
Dumbbell shoulder press	6-8	3
Dumbbell incline bench press	6-8	3
Lateral raise	12-15	3
Overhead triceps extension	12-15	3

DAY 2: PULL		
Exercise	Reps	Sets
Wide-grip pull-down/pull-up	6-8	3
Reverse fly or face pull	12-15	3
Straight-arm lat pull-down	12-15	3
Wide-grip shrug	12-15	3
Biceps curl	12-15	3

DAY 3: LOWER BODY		
Exercise	Reps	Sets
Standing calf raise	12-15	4
Squat	6-8	3
Romanian deadlift	6-8	3
Single-leg extension	12-15	3
Lying leg curl	12-15	3

DAY 4: UPPER BODY		
Exercise	Reps	Sets
Dumbbell shoulder press	6–8	3
Reverse/neutral-grip pull-up/ pull-down	6–8	3
Flat bench press	6–8	3
Wide-grip pull-down/pull-up	6–8	3
Upright row	12–15	3
Incline fly	12–15	3

DAY 5: LOWER BODY		
Exercise	Reps	Sets
Standing calf raise	12–15	4
Romanian deadlift	6–8	3
Squat	6–8	3
Seated leg curl	12–15	3
Single-leg extension	12–15	3
Overhead triceps extension	12–15	3
Hammer curl	12–15	3

Phase 1: The 4-Day Program

DAY 1: UPPER BODY 1		
Exercise	Reps	Sets
Flat bench press	6–8	3
Wide-grip pull-down/pull-up	6–8	3
Dumbbell shoulder press	6–8	3
Reverse-grip pull-down	6–8	3
Incline fly	12–15	3
Upright row	12–15	3

DAY 2: LOWER BODY 1		
Exercise	Reps	Sets
Standing calf raise	12–15	4
Squat	6–8	3
Romanian deadlift	6–8	3
Single-leg extension	12–15	3
Leg curl	12–15	3
Overhead triceps extension	12–15	3
Biceps curl	12–15	3

DAY 3: UPPER BODY 2		
Exercise	Reps	Sets
Wide-grip pull-down/pull-up	6–8	3
Dumbbell shoulder press	6–8	3
Flat bench press	6–8	3
Straight-arm lat pull-down	12–15	3

Exercise	Reps	Sets
Lateral raise	12–15	3
Incline bench press	12–15	3
Wide-grip shrug	12–15	3
Reverse fly	12–15	3

DAY 4: LOWER BODY 2

Exercise	Reps	Sets
Standing calf raise	12–15	4
Romanian deadlift	6–8	3
Squat	6–8	3
Leg curl	12–15	3
Single-leg extension	12–15	3
Overhead triceps extension	12–15	3
Hammer curl	12–15	3

Phase 1: The 3-Day Program

DAY 1: PUSH

Exercise	Reps	Sets
Flat bench press	6–8	3
Dumbbell shoulder press	6–8	3
Dumbbell incline bench press	6–8	3
Lateral raise	12–15	3
Overhead triceps extension	12–15	3

DAY 2: PULL

Exercise	Reps	Sets
Wide-grip pull-down/pull-up	6–8	3
Neutral-grip pull-down/pull-up	6–8	3
Upright row	12–15	3
Reverse fly or face pull	12–15	3
Wide-grip shrug	12–15	3
Biceps curl	12–15	3

DAY 3: LOWER BODY

Exercise	Reps	Sets
Standing calf raise	12–15	4
Squat	6–8	3
Romanian deadlift	6–8	3
Single-leg extension	12–15	3
Lying leg curl	12–15	3

PHASE 2 PROGRAMS

Phase 2: The 6-Day Program

DAY 1: PUSH—CHEST DOMINANT

Exercise	Reps	Sets
Flat bench press	6–8	4
Dumbbell shoulder press	6–8	4
Dumbbell incline bench press	6–8	4
Lateral raise	12–15	4
Overhead triceps extension	12–15	4

DAY 2: PULL—OUTER LAT DOMINANT

Exercise	Reps	Sets
Wide-grip pull-down/pull-up	6–8	4
Reverse fly or face pull	12–15	4
Straight-arm lat pull-down	12–15	4
Wide-grip shrug	12–15	4
Biceps curl	12–15	4

DAY 3: LOWER—QUAD DOMINANT

Exercise	Reps	Sets
Standing calf raise	12–15	5
Squat	6–8	4
Romanian deadlift	6–8	4
Single-leg extension	12–15	4
Lying leg curl	12–15	4

DAY 4: PUSH—SHOULDER DOMINANT

Exercise	Reps	Sets
Dumbbell shoulder press	6–8	4
Flat bench press	6–8	4
Lateral raise	12–15	4
Incline fly	12–15	4
Overhead triceps extension	12–15	4

DAY 5: PULL—INNER LAT DOMINANT

Exercise	Reps	Sets
Reverse/neutral-grip pull-up/pull-down	6–8	4
Upright row	12–15	4
Wide-grip pull-down/pull-up	6–8	4
Reverse fly or face pull	12–15	4
Hammer curl	12–15	4

DAY 6: LOWER BODY—HAMSTRING DOMINANT

Exercise	Reps	Sets
Standing calf raise	12–15	5
Romanian deadlift	6–8	4
Squat	6–8	4
Seated leg curl	12–15	4
Single-leg extension	12–15	4

Phase 2: The 5-Day Program

DAY 1: PUSH		
Exercise	Reps	Sets
Flat bench press	6–8	4
Dumbbell shoulder press	6–8	4
Dumbbell incline bench press	6–8	4
Lateral raise	12–15	4
Overhead triceps extension	12–15	4

DAY 2: PULL		
Exercise	Reps	Sets
Wide-grip pull-down/pull-up	6–8	4
Reverse fly or face pull	12–15	4
Straight-arm lat pulldown	12–15	4
Wide-grip shrug	12–15	4
Biceps curl	12–15	4

DAY 3: LOWER BODY		
Exercise	Reps	Sets
Standing calf raise	12–15	5
Squat	6–8	4
Romanian deadlift	6–8	3
Single-leg extension	12–15	3
Lying leg curl	12–15	3

DAY 4: UPPER BODY

Exercise	Reps	Sets
Dumbbell shoulder press	6–8	4
Reverse/neutral-grip pull-up/ pull-down	6–8	4
Flat bench press	6–8	4
Wide-grip pull-down/pull-up	6–8	4
Upright row	12–15	4
Incline fly	12–15	4

DAY 5: LOWER BODY

Exercise	Reps	Sets
Standing calf raise	12–15	5
Romanian deadlift	6–8	4
Squat	6–8	3
Seated leg curl	12–15	3
Single-leg extension	12–15	3
Overhead triceps extension	12–15	4
Hammer curl	12–15	4

Phase 2: The 4-Day Program

DAY 1: UPPER BODY 1		
Exercise	Reps	Sets
Flat bench press	6–8	4
Wide-grip pull-down/pull-up	6–8	4
Dumbbell shoulder press	6–8	4
Reverse-grip pull-down	6–8	4
Incline fly	12–15	4
Upright row	12–15	4

DAY 2: LOWER BODY 1		
Exercise	Reps	Sets
Standing calf raise	12–15	5
Squat	6–8	4
Romanian deadlift	6–8	4
Single-leg extension	12–15	4
Leg curl	12–15	4
Overhead triceps extension	12–15	4
Biceps curl	12–15	4

DAY 3: UPPER BODY 2		
Exercise	Reps	Sets
Wide-grip pull-down/pull-up	6–8	4
Dumbbell shoulder press	6–8	4
Flat bench press	6–8	4
Straight-arm lat pull-down	12–15	4

Exercise	Reps	Sets
Lateral raise	12–15	4
Incline bench press	12–15	4
Wide-grip shrug	12–15	4
Reverse fly	12–15	4

DAY 4: LOWER BODY 2

Exercise	Reps	Sets
Standing calf raise	12–15	5
Romanian deadlift	6–8	4
Squat	6–8	4
Leg curl	12–15	4
Single-leg extension	12–15	4
Overhead triceps extension	12–15	4
Hammer curl	12–15	4

Phase 2: The 3-Day Program

DAY 1: PUSH		
Exercise	**Reps**	**Sets**
Flat bench press	6–8	4
Dumbbell shoulder press	6–8	4
Dumbbell incline bench press	6–8	4
Lateral raise	12–15	4
Overhead triceps extension	12–15	4

DAY 2: PULL		
Exercise	**Reps**	**Sets**
Wide-grip pull-down/pull-up	6–8	4
Neutral-grip pull-down/pull-up	6–8	4
Upright row	12–15	4
Reverse fly or face pull	12–15	4
Wide-grip shrug	12–15	4
Biceps curl	12–15	4

DAY 3: LOWER BODY		
Exercise	**Reps**	**Sets**
Standing calf raise	12–15	4
Squat	6–8	4
Romanian deadlift	6–8	4
Single-leg extension	12–15	4
Lying leg curl	12–15	4

◇◇◇

I recommend that you try the *Physique Secrets* programs for at least a few months before deviating from the path and creating your own program.

Creating a high-quality strength-training program is not an easy task. You can go to the gym and move around some weights, do a ton of different exercises, and get a good workout. But that isn't training.

There are many things that work together that are often overlooked. Building the body you want takes a balanced approach with special consideration for each strength-training variable. You need to consider your training goals, training variables, recovery, diet, genetics, and more. The programs I've provided put all these and more into consideration.

If you are consistent, you should be able to build a good amount of beautiful muscle mass for at least the next year using the *Physique Secrets* program. Yes, you can stick with phase 2 for a year or more if you follow the proper progression model.

CHAPTER 26

IMPLEMENTING EXERCISE MANIPULATION

One of the biggest bodybuilding myths is the need to do a lot of slightly different exercises to stress the same muscle. This is interpreted as meaning you have to do a lot of different exercises for one specific muscle in a training session, or that you need to switch up your program often with different exercises.

This myth leads to the mistake of switching exercises before obtaining maximal benefits. It also means that your neuromuscular system has to restart and learn a new movement pattern before you can optimally stress each of the muscle fibers.

The truth is, exercise manipulation isn't nearly as important as it is made out to be. Having said that, it is important to have the correct exercises to start with in your program. After all, they are the vehicles for transferring gravitational force into muscular tension.

Also, being able to change your exercises is important for continuing to build muscle and strength, but knowing when to change exercises and how to change to new but similar exercises without losing the muscle and strength you've already built can be hard to do.

If the core exercises you started with are working for you or you can't change your equipment, then this chapter isn't necessary for you at this point. It would be more beneficial to skip to the next chapter and implement progressive overload.

It's important to understand that when I say "exercise manipulation," I don't mean that you have to know fancy techniques, have an advanced knowledge of anatomy, or do anything out of the ordinary. What I mean is being able to determine which muscle you want to train, understanding how it functions, and selecting exercises that stress its movement pattern. Then you can choose the exercises that will best help you achieve your goals, and make your final choice based on the equipment you have, the time you have, any injuries you have, and your anatomical structure. Basically, manipulating your exercises to fit you, your program, and your goals.

Exercise manipulation is a vast topic that can get very confusing very quickly. For this reason, I will only give you specific recommendations for how to adjust the exercises of the *Physique Secrets* programs to better fit your situation and goals.

You can also refer back to the previous chapters where we discussed the different muscle groups, how your muscles function, and the top exercises.

HOW TO ADJUST THE EXERCISES IN THE *PHYSIQUE SECRETS* PROGRAMS

When creating the *Physique Secrets* programs, I purposefully selected exercises that would require very little equipment. Sure, having enough weight to add to a barbell or having heavy enough dumbbells will be a key factor in getting stronger and continuing to improve, but overall, you won't need any fancy equipment to complete the program and achieve an incredible body.

If you do have to adjust exercises due to limited equipment or minor injuries, try to keep the same exercise but use different equipment. You want to have the same movement pattern and muscles trained—or be as close as possible.

You also want to maintain the same stress provided to your body. If the program calls for a heavy compound or multi-joint exercise, you will want to do another heavy compound or multi-joint exercise.

If you can't perform the same exercise and movement due to limited equipment or injuries, you can add exercises that train the same muscles but with equipment that you have available. You can use the exercises mentioned in the muscle group analysis chapter.

You can also swap barbells for dumbbells or cables, adjust your grip or the handle used during training to help with injuries, or use bands or body-weight exercises if you don't have any equipment at all.

As long as you keep the same fundamental movement, you'll be fine for now.

Here are some options for switching exercises:

EXERCISE	ALTERNATES
Squat	Front or back squat, normal or wide stance, high bar or low bar, Bulgarian split squat, reverse lunge
Wide-grip pull-up/pull-down	Assisted pull-up machine, band-assisted pull-up, neutral grip, reverse grip, single arm
Dumbbell shoulder press	Barbell military press
Romanian deadlift	Pull-through, hip extension, dumbbells or barbell, single leg
Bench press	Barbell, dumbbells, incline barbell or dumbbells, cable/dumbbell fly, weighted push-up, close grip
Straight-arm lat pull-down	Machine, cable, dumbbells, bent/EZ bar, kneeling, different cable attachments, lat prayer

Standing calf raise	Seated calf raise, donkey calf raise, single leg
Lateral raise	Dumbbells, cable, machine, upright row with bar/dumbbells/cable, butterfly raise
Upright row	Dumbbells, barbell, cable machine, bent/EZ bar, lateral raise, butterfly raise, shoulder press
Leg extension	Single leg, machine, cable, sissy squat
Leg curl	Seated, lying, single leg, standing, machine, cable, glute-ham raise
Reverse fly or face pull	Cable, machine, single arm, dumbbell bent-over, barbell or dumbbell high chest row
Wide-grip shrug	Barbell, single arm, cable, dumbbells, hex bar, shrug machine, calf-raise machine
Overhead triceps extension	Cable, machine, dumbbells, single arm, skullcrusher, bent/EZ bar
Single-arm biceps curl	Cable facing away, cable facing machine, dumbbell, machine, barbell, hammer curl

AD LIBITUM ABDOMINAL WORK

If you've looked through or are following the *Physique Secrets* training program, you probably noticed that it doesn't have any abdominal-specific work. We talked about why this is the case when we first looked at the five key exercises, so if you need a refresher, go back to that chapter.

Still, for those who either want to or feel they need to develop their midsection a bit more, I have created two ab circuits for you. They probably look very simple to most people who have done core training before—and that's because they are.

These example routines can be done two or three times a week as needed. You can also split up each routine into six total days by doing one exercise a day for three days and then repeating. This option would help keep down your time in the gym each day.

EXAMPLE AB WORKOUT 1 (LIGHT WEIGHT)		
Exercise	Reps	Sets
Plank (side and regular)	1 minute	2–3
Bosu-ball or exercise-ball crunch	20+	2

Lying reverse crunch	20+	2
Oblique twist with a light wood bar on the shoulders/traps	30+	2

EXAMPLE AB WORKOUT 2 (HEAVY WEIGHT)

Exercise	Reps	Sets
Weighted or cable crunch	12–20	3
Oblique twist with cable machine	20–30	3
Hanging reverse crunch	20+	3

ADJUSTING THE ORDER OF EXERCISES

Adjust the order of exercises based on the results you want to achieve and the muscles or exercises you want to prioritize. Exercise order is important for ensuring body and strength symmetry while also ensuring that you provide the maximum effort for the most important and difficult exercises.

The exercises in the *Physique Secrets* programs are ordered so that the heavier, more technically difficult, and larger-muscle-group exercises are first in each training session. They then work backward in intensity, difficulty, and size of muscle groups.

However, there are a few ways that you can adjust the order of exercises based on which muscles and exercises you want to prioritize, to prevent boredom, or to improve your body's symmetry.

First, you can adjust the order by beginning each workout with the exercises that you hope will give you the best chance of increasing in strength where you want it. Or you can do first the exercises that train muscles you want to give the best chance for maximal growth.

For example, you can do shoulder presses before bench presses to aim for the best results for your shoulders as opposed to your chest.

However, it's important that you only switch the order of exercises that use the same-size muscle groups and are of similar difficulty. Don't do leg extensions before squats, for example, or biceps curls before shoulder presses.

If you want to prevent possible boredom and enhance muscle strength and symmetry, you can adjust your exercise order by switching back and forth between two exercises to provide the same stress with each.

For example, you can start one training session with the flat bench press, followed by the shoulder press. Then, in your next training session, you could switch it up by doing the shoulder press first, and then the incline bench press.

You can adjust your exercise order either after every training session or monthly. Changing your exercise order every training session simply provides you with two different (but similar) training days. This allows you to progress with each program.

SECRET 9

–

CREATING A BODY-TRANSFORMING NUTRITION PROGRAM

CHAPTER 27

INTRODUCTION TO MEAL PLAN CONSTRUCTION

Succeeding with dieting takes a different approach from the one we used for strength training. Here, slowly implementing the different variables in stages will have the opposite effect than it does for training.

Dieting has too many interrelated factors. Yes, there is still an order of importance, especially when making a meal plan, but putting the different parts of a diet into place in this order ignores what makes dieting so hard. It fails to account for the psychological aspects, hunger, cravings, diet sustainability, and pressure from society, friends, and family.

For example, say you start by just trying to eat the correct number of calories each day without worrying about nutrient content or having any real structure. You could unknowingly eat all your allotted calories for the day in one large breakfast.

Sure, you hit your target, but your protein intake might have been incredibly low, and the rest of the day is going to be a struggle.

Instead, a diet needs to be implemented in a manner that helps you accurately determine the calories and macronutrients you eat, create a basic meal plan that works for you, bridge the gap between the results you want as quickly as possible and the amount of time and effort required, and finally, keep making progress for life because you created a solid foundation to build on.

In this section, we will go over all of that in a way that allows you to finally get results and put the stresses of dieting behind you.

To begin, we'll look at the factors you need to consider when determining what you want out of your diet compared with what you're willing to do. This will tell you what to focus on based on your goals, lifestyle, previous dieting experience, preferences, and current body.

Next, we'll go over step-by-step how to easily create a meal plan. By drawing up a basic meal plan based on your schedule, food preferences, calories, and macronutrients, you will be able to take the all-important first steps.

This is where most people fail. They have their meal plan in hand or have written down a few recipes they want to try, but overwhelm sets in. They don't know what to do next, whether their meal plan is good enough, or how to track and measure everything to ensure results.

So, once we've created your meal plan, we'll go over exactly what you need to do at the very beginning to set yourself on the path to success now and in the future.

If you follow everything we discuss throughout this section and put it into practice, you will lay the perfect foundation for rapid body transformation and sustainable dieting. All you'll have to do is make slight adjustments to your program, add in supplements, and slowly work toward not needing to diet or track everything you eat—all of which we'll discuss in Part VI.

CHAPTER 28

YOUR TARGETS FOR FLEXIBLE DIETING SUCCESS

In chapter 9, in the section on dieting variables, we discussed the four guidelines for flexible dieting success. As a quick recap, they were:

Balance your physique goals with what is realistic for your diet adherence, lifestyle, experience, and preferences.

1. Prioritize calorie quantity over quality.

2. Eat enough high-quality protein every single day.

3. Compose at least 75% of your diet from satiating plant-based, nutrient-dense, whole foods and lean complete protein sources.

4. These guidelines help you see that dieting success doesn't need to be nearly as restrictive as a lot of people are led to believe. The four precepts also show you what to concentrate on in creating a meal plan and in day-to-day dieting.

It's all about structure and balance with a flexible mindset. When applying the different nutrition variables, how you structure and balance your meal plan will determine your dieting consistency and the amount of tracking you might need to do to get results.

So, in order to create the best diet, structure the diet so it fits your schedule and meal preferences. This will help you form a routine and solid eating habits.

Then add a balance of different food groups with a variety of different food sources that can easily be mixed and matched to prevent monotony and increase diet quality.

However, to put the dieting guidelines and approach into practice so that you build an amazing physique, you need to eat the correct calories and nutrients for simultaneous fat loss and muscle building.

This doesn't just happen by chance. It requires tracking what you eat to be certain you're doing everything correctly.

Tracking calories and macronutrients has been shown to be the most effective and rapid way to get results, but it is also not sustainable for a lot of people. It can be more effort than you're willing to put in and can lead to a stricter diet than you want.

So, when it comes to tracking your food and implementing everything, it's important to consider the results you want and the amount of accuracy and consistency required to get you there.

RESULTS AND ACCURACY AND CONSISTENCY (OH MY)

Assuming you have a structured, balanced, and flexible meal plan in place, and you understand how to adjust foods and track your calories and macros (which we'll cover in an upcoming chapter), the goal should be to turn dieting into a lifestyle and get long-term results.

To do this, you want to be only as accurate as needed in order to be consistent enough to get the results you want.

The more accurate and strict you are with your calories and nutrients, the more consistent your results will be, but your long-term dieting consistency and sustainability will suffer.

The less accurate and more flexible you are with what you eat, the less consistent your results will be, but you will be able to stay consistent with this diet for longer.

It's a sliding scale of consistency between accurate tracking, diet strictness, and rapid results on one side and no tracking, complete flexibility to eat what you want, and no results on the other.

Your goals, current physique, and desired timeline for results will determine how strict and precise you need to be with your calories and macronutrients versus how relaxed your eating and tracking can be. Both will determine the amount of dieting consistency needed and the length of time during which you can maintain this consistency.

For example, a person who wants to cut down from 10% body fat to 7% body fat will need to be far more accurate and strict, but for a shorter time than a person who just wants to lose 30 pounds in a year.

Then, once the cut has been made, the accuracy and strictness will need to be adjusted to avoid diet failure and gaining the weight back, and ensure long-term consistency.

To help you match your precision with your needs, there are tracking targets to aim for.

YOUR BASIC TRACKING TARGETS

I want to break this down for you so it makes sense and is easy to follow.

For the best short-term results, you need to be very accurate, strict, and consistent with your calorie and macronutrient intakes.

For the best long-term results, you should track as little as you need, allow for flexibility, and be consistent with your dietary structure and balance.

Those are the boundaries for results. Any combination in between is your choice, although I'll offer some recommendations based on certain situations.

If all that makes sense, let's lay out the tracking targets for you to aim for and when you might use each one.

When aiming for a target, there will be times when you aren't able to hit the target due to social events, stress, work, travel, and so on. When this happens, maintain a flexible mindset and aim for the next-closest target, or just try to stay as close as possible.

Just because you miss a target doesn't mean the day is a waste and you can or should use it as a free-for-all.

The Closest Target

What to aim for:

- Being within +/-200 calories or +/-10% of the prescribed calories, whichever is closer to your target calories

This target is not for food-tracking beginners, except when the other targets were missed. Instead, it's best for people who:

- Have a basic feel for calories and macros from experience.

- Want a relaxed diet and have experience tracking their food.

- Have a busy lifestyle.

- Have a medium to low body fat percentage.

The Middle Target

What to aim for:

- Being within +/-10 grams of your daily protein requirement

- Being within +/-200 calories or +/-10% of the prescribed calories, whichever is closer to your target calories

- A diet with at least 75% whole foods, a variety of fruits and vegetables, and mostly healthy fats

The middle target is where you will probably spend most of your fitness and nutrition journey. It is accurate enough to keep getting you results but doesn't require excessive tracking of your calories and all the macronutrients.

If you establish a structured and balanced meal plan, you should be able to hit these targets consistently and maintain a long-term diet. This can also help you get to the point of not tracking anything and instead using intuition and your natural hunger to determine accuracy, though this should be later rather than sooner.

This target is ideal for:

- The average gym-goer and strength trainee.

- People who are at a higher body fat percentage or are dieting for the first time (and thus need time to establish habits and experience).

- People who struggle with dieting and getting results.

- Maintenance dieters.

- People above 10%–12% body fat.

The Farthest Target

What to aim for:

- Being within +/-5 grams of your daily protein requirement

- Being within +/-100 calories or +/-5% of the prescribed calories, whichever is closer to your target calories

- Being within +/-10 grams of your dietary fat target and +/-20 grams of your carb target; exact ratio isn't important

- A diet with at least 75% whole foods, a variety of fruits and vegetables, and mostly healthy fats

- 35 grams of fiber daily and increased omega-3 fatty acid intake

- Because this is the farthest target away from you, hitting it will mean you need to be very accurate with your calorie and macronutrient intakes and maintain more consistency with what you eat. You'll need to make sure your diet is structured and well balanced so that you can meet your targets, get enough micronutrients, and curb your hunger with foods that fill you up.

This target isn't ideal for long periods of time but can be great for getting back on track with your meal plan, checking to make sure you're doing things correctly, breaking plateaus, or making little cuts when needed.

As such, this target is ideal for:

- The short term.

- Serious strength trainees who have already built a good amount of muscle.

- People advanced enough to track their food intake with high accuracy.

- Dieters who are able to ignore internal cues like hunger when those signals don't match external cues like the number of calories in a serving of food.

- Trainees who are at or below 10%–12% body fat and are cutting to single-digit levels.

◇◇◇

In the next chapter, we'll create a meal plan that will provide you with a structured eating schedule and a balance of foods. After your first two weeks on this meal plan, in which you will train yourself to track your food properly, you should move into one of the three tracking targets we just discussed.

You don't need to track everything you eat once you become experienced enough with registering how hungry your body is, how well you're improving in the gym, how your body weight and composition are fluctuating, and then how to adjust your food intake to either keep seeing results or get yourself back on track.

However, you first need to gain experience. Plus, who knows, a lot of people prefer to track their food as a way to stay motivated.

CHAPTER 29

HOW TO EASILY CREATE A MEAL PLAN STEP-BY-STEP FROM SCRATCH

Having the proper dieting strategy, understanding the different variables that make up a diet, slowly learning through real-world implementation, and making adjustments based on the results you're getting will provide you with a majority of what you need to transform your body and life.

Creating a basic meal plan to provide structure and ensure that you have a balanced diet is an important practice. This is especially true if you are just starting out, have had dieting struggles in the past, or need a high level of diet precision.

Too many strength trainees rely on premade meal plans devised for the mass market and never learn how to actually create one for themselves, based on what they need to succeed now and in the future. A premade plan might seem like the easier option, but that's only because coming up with your own meal plan has the reputation of being a time-consuming, headache-inducing process.

Instead, a meal plan should provide an outline that you can use to guide your everyday eating habits and dieting routine. It shouldn't be a strict program that has everything calculated down to the last calorie without any wiggle room or adjustments allowed.

There are too many factors involved to even create a perfect meal plan on paper.

In this chapter, I want to put your mind at ease by taking you through the process of creating a meal plan from scratch, step-by-step. Once you see it all together and understand how each piece works to create a final meal plan, you can simply plug in your numbers and follow the steps here.

Whenever you are creating a meal plan from scratch, I highly recommend that you come back to this chapter to follow the steps with ease and speed.

Now, let's get into the exact steps you need to follow to create a complete program from scratch.

MEAL PLAN CREATION STEPS

For the best results, each step in creating a meal plan needs to be done in a specific order. At first it might seem like a lot of information, but as you progress from one step to the next, you'll realize it's far easier than many people think.

Here are the exact steps we'll take to ensure that your meal plan is the best it can be:

1. Determine optimal daily calorie intake based on weight goals.

2. Determine grams of each macronutrient to eat daily.

3. Create your eating schedule, determine meals, and note recipes.

4. Add protein sources to your meal plan.

5. Add fruits and vegetables, followed by other carbohydrate sources.

6. Add healthy dietary fats to create complete meals.

7. Fill in calorie and macronutrient gaps to create real meals while ensuring sustainability and enjoyment.

Using this step-by-step method, you will be able to create an enjoyable and body-transforming nutrition program. Past dieting troubles don't dictate your future dieting successes. You've got this!

STEP #1: DETERMINE OPTIMAL DAILY CALORIE INTAKE BASED ON WEIGHT GOALS

Necessary variables for calculations:

*   Your weight in pounds or kilograms

*   Your height in inches or meters

*   Your current age in years

*   Your activity factor based on your daily and weekly activity and training level

*   Your cutting or bulking factor based on the percentage of maintenance calories you'll be consuming

Step #1.1: Determine Your Resting Energy Expenditure (REE)

REE (calories) = 5.45 × (weight in pounds) + 15 × (height in inches) - 8.16 × (age in years) + 216

REE (calories) = 12 × (weight in kilograms) + 590.4 × (height in meters) - 8.16 × (age in years) + 216

Example:

Step #1.2: Determine Your Total Daily Energy Expenditure (TDEE)

TDEE = REE × activity factor

ACTIVITY FACTOR (AF) TABLE

Level of Activity	Weekly Activity	Activity Factor (AF) Adjustment
Sedentary	Little or no exercise and a desk job	1.2
Lightly Active	Trains 1 to 3 days per week	1.35
Moderately Active	Trains 4 or 5 days per week	1.5
Very Active	Trains 6 or 7 days per week	1.7
Extremely Active	Very heavy exercise or a physical job or trains twice per day	1.85

Step #1.3: Determine Optimal Calorie Intake for Weight-Change Goals

Optimal weight-loss calorie intake = TDEE × (1 - optimal deficit %)

Optimal weight-gain calorie intake = TDEE × (1 + initial energy surplus %)

Optimal maintenance calorie intake = (body weight) × (maintenance calorie factor)

WEIGHT-CHANGE TABLE

Body Fat Percentage	Optimal Weight Change
Above 12%	20%-25% calorie deficit
Going from 12% to 7%-8%	10% calorie deficit
Maintaining 7%-9%	TDEE
Bulking under 12%	5%-10% calorie surplus

MAINTENANCE CALORIE FACTORS

Workouts per week	3 or 4 (Beginner)	5 or More (Experienced)
Calories/lb of body weight	15	19
Calories/kg of body weight	33	42

STEP #2: DETERMINE MACRONUTRIENT REQUIREMENTS

Step #2.1: Determine Your Protein Needs and Calculate Calories from Protein

Daily protein intake in grams = body weight in pounds × 0.82 g/lb

Daily protein intake in grams = body weight in kilograms × 1.8 g/kg

Daily protein intake in calories = grams of protein × 4 calories per gram

Step #2.2: Determine Your Fat Intake and Calculate Calories from Fat

> Daily fat intake in calories = cutting or bulking calories × 0.3

> Daily fat intake in grams = calories of fat / 9 calories per gram

Step #2.3: Determine Your Carbohydrate Intake Based on Remaining Calories

> Daily carb intake in calories = total daily calories – protein calories – fat calories

> Target grams of carbohydrates = carbohydrate target calories / 4 calories per gram

STEP #3: DETERMINE MEAL PLAN STRUCTURE

Step #3.1: Determine Your Ideal Meal and Nutrient Timing

Based on your normal daily schedule, hunger, and workout times, determine the number of meals you will eat and when you should eat them. Your meal timing should be simple, aside from eating 30 to 40 grams of protein, most likely in a complete meal, within 2 hours pre-workout and again post-workout.

Step #3.2: Split Your Macronutrients between Your Meals

It's time to finalize your eating schedule and the approximate number of macronutrients you'll consume at each meal. As long as your calorie and protein intakes are close to what they should be, the exact numbers of calories, carbs, fats, and proteins don't need to be perfect.

For ease, split your macronutrients evenly based on your number of meals:

> Protein per meal = daily protein intake / number of meals

> Carbs per meal = daily carb intake / number of meals

> Fats per meal = daily fat intake / number of meals

It's important to understand that you don't need to stress about having everything perfect. The little details are insignificant to your long-term results, and everything can be changed.

Having a few grams of carbs or fat missing, not getting the nutritionists' recommended five to six daily servings of fruits and veggies, or eating your pre-workout meal 4 hours before your workout won't make or break your results.

Step #3.3: Determine Possible Meals and Make a List of Recipes

As you are finalizing your eating schedule, you need to make a note of possible meals you can make and their recipes. Knowing what you'll eat for each meal will make plugging in actual food and serving sizes much easier. And having recipes that you would like to try or make regularly will allow you to know which foods you'll need to add to your meal plan and roughly how many servings of each.

When looking for recipes or determining meals, make sure they're healthy, simple, and quick and easy to make, and that they don't require a lot of extra calories added. If your recipe calls for a lot of butter to be added for taste, it's most likely not the best option to include.

However, you can always switch unhealthy options for healthier ones and adjust serving sizes. For example, if your recipe calls for butter, you can try using extra virgin olive oil instead. Another example is using brown rice or quinoa instead of white rice, or whole wheat bread instead of white bread.

To switch serving sizes, you can increase the healthy parts of the meal and recipe while decreasing the unhealthy parts. For instance, you can easily increase vegetables and fruits while using less of the high-calorie carb source in your recipe. This could be making a larger salad, then having a smaller serving of spaghetti.

For now, taking note of the different meals you'll eat and recipes you'll enjoy, and understanding that they can be changed easily, will be all you need to complete this step.

Personally, I stick to a very simple diet layout:

> **Meal 1: fruit-and-veggie smoothie with protein powder**
> **Workout**
> **Meal 2: sandwich, Greek yogurt, fruit, other protein source as needed (usually hard-boiled eggs)**
> **Meal 3: hearty meat source; cooked vegetables or salad; carb source like rice, pasta, or potatoes**

STEP #4: ADD PROTEIN SOURCES

Since protein is vitally important for muscle building and satiety, you will add it to your diet first. To help you understand, I've separated the different food groups into specific serving sizes with similar nutritional makeups.

All of the food source tables in steps #4 through 6 were created to get you started by providing you with a simple-to-use format for creating a meal plan. The foods listed can be used as healthy foods to include in your daily meals, and each of their macronutrient profiles is a fairly accurate estimate that will help you get a meal plan foundation in place.

However, you'll still need to dial in the calories and precise macronutrients based on the weight and nutrition facts of the foods you have available—which is done in step #7.

Like the rest of the book, creating a foundation to build on is important and will make your life much easier when you put everything into practice.

To plan your meals in this way, follow the steps below for each macronutrient:

1.   Determine what food you want for each meal.

2.   Determine how many servings of a food source you need to meet your protein intake requirement for each meal.

3.   Take the number of servings of a food source and multiply it by the size of the serving to get how much of each food item you should eat.

4.   Mix and match foods and servings of foods until you hit your grams of protein and have a good start to a legitimate meal.

For example, a single serving of a lean protein source will have 7 grams of protein, zero grams of carbohydrates, and zero to 3 grams of fat, accounting for 35 to 55 calories. Therefore, if your meal plan calls for 28 grams of protein for a meal, you can figure on four servings of lean protein. Another option is having three servings of lean protein and one serving of medium-fat protein.

So, if you want a sandwich with turkey and cheese and you need 35 grams of protein in this meal, you will have three servings of turkey and two servings of cheese. This will be 3 ounces of turkey and 2 ounces of cheese, since the tables show that both turkey and cheese have a serving size of 1 ounce.

Protein Food Sources

The protein sources below are just a few of the foods you can incorporate in your meal plan to help with your muscle-building and fat-loss journey. There are several other sources you can substitute. What I've provided here isn't mandatory for perfect health; you can include any other food that you love.

Lean Protein	Portion Size	Carbs (g)	Protein (g)	Fat (g)
Skinless white-meat poultry	1 oz (30 g)	-	7	1
Skinless dark-meat poultry or white-meat chicken with skin	1 oz (30 g)	-	7	3
Egg whites	2 count	-	7	1
Lean beef, pork, lamb	1 oz (30 g)	-	7	3
Cheese	1 oz (30 g)	-	7	3
Beans, peas, lentils	½ cup (100 g)	-	7	1
White fish	1 oz (30 g)	-	7	1
Tuna	1 oz (30 g)	-	7	1
Oysters, salmon, catfish, sardines	1 oz (30 g)	-	7	3
All shellfish	1 oz (30 g)	-	7	1

Medium-Fat Protein	Portion Size	Carbs (g)	Protein (g)	Fat (g)
Most beef, pork, lamb, and dark-meat poultry with skin	1 oz (30 g)	-	7	5
Whole egg	1 count	-	7	5
Fattier cheese	1 oz (30 g)	-	7	5
Cottage cheese	¼ cup (56 g)	-	7	5
Tofu	4 oz or ½ cup (120 g)	-	7	5

Milk and Yogurt	Portion Size	Carbs (g)	Protein (g)	Fat (g)
Nonfat milk	1 cup (240 ml)	12	8	0
Low-fat milk	1 cup (240 ml)	12	8	3

Plain nonfat yogurt	1 cup (230 g)	12	8	0
Plain nonfat Greek yogurt	6 oz (173 g)	12	8	0

STEP #5: ADD HEALTHY CARBOHYDRATES

Since carbohydrates are your primary source of vitamins and minerals and your only source of fiber, it is essential to ensure that you place whole food sources first before added carbohydrates (processed) or other foods.

For starters, place your fruits and vegetables into your program, followed by whole grains and legumes (beans), and finish with any other form of carbohydrate as a filler after most of the plan is already created.

Remember, our primary goal is health, which means you will first want to hit your fiber, vitamin, and mineral needs before anything else. The more whole foods you eat that contain fiber, the more satiating the food will be, and the more calories your body will burn digesting the food.

So, by starting with whole carbohydrates, you can improve your health and help with fat loss at the same time.

Try to hit 75%–80% of your determined carb intake with healthy carbs. This will allow for optimal health, fat loss, muscle building, and satiety while also including some carbohydrate servings or added calories for when you get hungry and want to eat extra for a meal, enjoy a snack, or indulge in dessert.

To figure out how many carbohydrates you need, use the tables below and the same method we used for proteins.

Fruits

Add as many fruits as possible. Fruits are high in nutrients, water, and fiber, which help boost your fullness. This helps prevent overeating, which, in turn, helps with fat loss.

Below is a list of common fruits.

Fruits	Portion Size	Carbs (g)	Protein (g)	Fat (g)
Most fruits	1 medium	15	-	-
Apple	1 medium	15	-	-
Asian pear	1 medium	15	-	-
Banana	1 small	15	-	-
Blackberries	¾ cup (80 g)	15	-	-

Blueberries	¾ cup (80 g)	15	-	-
Cantaloupe	1 cup (156 g)	15	-	-
Cherries	¾ cup (80 g)	15	-	-
Grapefruit	½ fruit	15	-	-
Grapes	¾ cup (80 g)	15	-	-
Kiwi	1 medium	15	-	-
Melons of any kind, diced	1 cup (156 g)	15	-	-
Nectarine	1 medium	15	-	-
Orange	1 medium	15	-	-
Peach	1 medium	15	-	-
Pear	1 medium	15	-	-
Pineapple	1 cup (156 g)	15	-	-
Raspberries	¾ cup (80 g)	15	-	-
Strawberries	1¼ cup (180 g)	15	-	-
Watermelon	1 cup (156 g)	15	-	-

Vegetables

Add as many vegetables as possible.

Vegetables	Portion Size	Carbs (g)	Protein (g)	Fat (g)
Most cooked vegetables	½ cup (81 g)	5	-	-
Most raw vegetables	1 cup (30–100 g)	5	-	-
Asparagus	See top of table	5	-	-
Bell pepper	See top of table	5	-	-

Broccoli	See top of table	5	-	-
Brussels sprouts	See top of table	5	-	-
Cauliflower	See top of table	5	-	-
Cucumber	See top of table	5	-	-
Eggplant	See top of table	5	-	-
Green beans	See top of table	5	-	-
Kale	See top of table	5	-	-
Mixed green salad	See top of table	5	-	-
Mushrooms	See top of table	5	-	-
Onion	See top of table	5	-	-
Spinach	See top of table	5	-	-
Zucchini	See top of table	5	-	-

Bread, Grains, and Starches

To maximize the health benefits of your nutrition plan, look for bread and grains with a fiber-to-to-tal-carbohydrate ratio of at least 1:4.

Breads, Grains, and Starches	Portion Size	Carbs (g)	Protein (g)	Fat (g)
Any beans or lentils	½ cup (100 g)	15	7	-
Bagel, English muffin, roll, or bun (whole wheat preferred)	1 count	30	-	-
Black beans	½ cup (100 g)	15	7	-
Brown rice	½ cup cooked (97 g)	15	-	-
Cereal	½ cup (15 g)	15	-	-
Ezekiel bread	1 slice	15	-	-
Granola	½ cup (30 g)	15	-	-

Most bread	1 slice	15	-	-
Oatmeal	½ cup (119 g)	15	-	-
Potato or sweet potato	1 small	15	-	-
Quinoa	½ cup cooked (97 g)	15	-	-
Rice cakes	2 count	15	-	-
Tortilla or pita	1 count (small)	15	-	-
Whole wheat bread	1 slice	15	-	-
Whole wheat pasta	½ cup cooked (97 g)	15	-	-

STEP #6: ADD HEALTHY DIETARY FATS

We'll use the same approach for fats as we did for protein: plugging in food-group servings followed by fat sources. As a reminder, you will take the different nutrients per food group, place them throughout your diet, and then fill in those nutrient servings with the number of servings of fat.

A single serving of a fat source will have 5 grams of fat, zero grams of carbohydrates, and zero grams of protein. This correlates to 45 calories (5 grams x 9 calories/gram = 45 calories).

If your meal plan calls for 15 grams of fat for a meal, you need three servings of a fat source. The other option is to get two servings from a fat source and one to two servings from a food group containing fat.

Below is a table of different fat sources and the size of a portion of each. I will remind you that these sources are just examples. The fact that I've selected them doesn't mean they are a must for perfect health. You could include any food that you love in your meal plan.

Unsaturated Fats

Monounsaturated and polyunsaturated fats are usually liquid at room temperature. These should be consumed in higher amounts than saturated fats.

Unsaturated Fats	Portion Size	Carbs (g)	Protein (g)	Fat (g)
Avocado	⅛ medium (2 Tbsp, 30 g)	-	-	5
Canola oil	1 tsp (5 g)	-	-	5
Corn oil	1 tsp (5 g)	-	-	5

Extra virgin olive oil	1 tsp (5 g)	-	-	5
Fatty fish like salmon and mackerel	1 oz (30 g)	-	7	3
Most nuts	6–10 count (9 g)	-	-	5
Most seeds	1 Tbsp (9 g)	-	-	5
Peanut oil	1 tsp (5 g)	-	-	5
Safflower oil	1 tsp (5 g)	-	-	5
Shellfish	1 oz (30 g)	-	7	1
Soybean oil	1 tsp (5 g)	-	-	5
Walnut oil	1 tsp (5 g)	-	-	5

Saturated Fats

Saturated fats are often solid at room temperature. Limit your intake of these to no more than 10% of your total calorie intake.

Saturated Fats	Portion Size	Carbs (g)	Protein (g)	Fat (g)
Butter and margarine	1 tsp (5 g)	-	-	5
Cheese	1 oz (30 g)	-	7	3
Creamer	1 Tbsp (15 g)	-	-	5
Egg yolks	1 count	-	4	4
Lard, palm oil, coconut oil	1 tsp (5 g)	-	-	5
Most animal proteins	See protein tables	-	-	-
Peanut butter and other nut butters	½ Tbsp (8 g)	-	-	5
Processed foods and desserts	Unknown	-	-	-
Whole milk	1 cup (240 ml)	12	8	8

STEP #7: MAKE MEALS, COMPLETE RECIPES, ENSURE SUSTAINABILITY

At this point, you will have almost a full meal plan in hand. You should have the correct amount of protein and at least 75%–80% of the correct amounts of healthy carbs and fats determined.

In the previous steps, you mapped out a structure for eating and fulfilled your necessary muscle-building and optimal health nutrients with their respective food sources. Now it's time to make minor adjustments to ensure that you can create actual meals with the foods you selected, and to make any adjustments to your plan to allow for flexibility, sustainability, and enjoyment.

Again, keep in mind that the food source tables are average estimates of macronutrient profiles of common foods. The food you have available in your fridge or pantry might have a completely different nutrient profile than you planned for and marked down. Simply make a note of this and you can fix any inaccuracies when you start actually weighing and measuring each food—which we'll discuss in the next chapter.

For now, the goal is to fill in any gaps that you see in your meal plan. To do this:

- Add, subtract, or rearrange foods to create real meals.

- Note recipes you want to try and the foods you need for the recipes.

- Adjust recipes to make them healthier and fit your macros.

- If you won't eat a specific food, get rid of it.

- Create alternative food options for your meals to keep to your structure but add flexibility.

- Add in a daily 100-to-200-calorie buffer for miscalculations, a large meal at the end of the week, or an unexpected social event.

- Add in low-calorie food alternatives and snacks to increase meal volume and reduce cravings.

- Reduce the variety of foods you consume in a meal to include one high-protein source and a satiating carb source, then use fats for flavor.

If you added a macronutrient source to hit a specific intake, then you might need to subtract a food source from one meal and increase the intake in another meal.

For example, maybe you added a random scoop of peanut butter to your breakfast plan. If you're not using it on toast or have no other use for it, you can eliminate it and replace it with avocado or olive oil for lunch or dinner.

Next, look through the list of recipes that you made in step 3. Arrange your food and ingredients to follow different recipes you might enjoy. This little spice of life will add a structured variety to your meal plan.

Finally, add in low-calorie snacks, small desserts, seasonings, and toppings. These add some flavor and help reduce cravings if your diet doesn't turn out to be satiating enough.

One of the easiest ways to stick to your diet is to swap high-calorie foods for lower-calorie alternatives. This could be rice cakes instead of chips, low-calorie sweeteners instead of sugar, oils instead of butter, and so on.

There are a ton of options; you just need to find what works for you, your budget, and your meal plan.

In the end, no meal plan is perfect. You just need to get started and test different things until you find enjoyable meals and recipes that also get you results.

HOW TO DO STEPS #1 THROUGH 3 FOR AN AVERAGE MAN

Here is a realistic example using a profile similar to that of the average American man. We'll look at a 30-year-old—let's call him Fred—who is 5'9" tall and weighs 200 pounds.

Let's assume Fred is well above 12% body fat and will therefore start by performing a cut. He trains five days a week using heavy weights and 16 sets per muscle per week. He eats three meals a day and trains in the afternoon.

So, his necessary variables for calculations are:

- Weight = 200 pounds

- Height = 69 inches

- Age = 30 years

- Activity factor = moderately active = 1.5

- Cutting factor = 25% deficit, or 0.75 of maintenance calories

Step #1: Determine Optimal Daily Calorie Intake Based on Weight Goals

- Resting energy expenditure = $5.45 \times (200) + 15 \times (69) - 8.16 \times (30) + 216$

- REE = 1,090 + 1,035 - 245 + 216 = 2,096 calories resting

- Total daily energy expenditure = $2,096 \times 1.5$

- TDEE = 3,144 calories burned daily on average

- Optimal daily calories = 3,144 × 0.75

- Optimal daily calories = 2,358 calories daily

Step #2: Determine Macronutrient Requirements

- Daily protein intake in grams = 200 × 0.82 = 164 grams of protein per day

- Daily protein intake in calories = 164 × 4 = 656 calories from protein

- Daily fat intake in calories = 2,358 × 0.3 = 707 calories from dietary fat

- Daily fat intake in grams = 707 / 9 = 78 grams of dietary fat per day (rounded down from 78.6 grams to prevent eating extra calories; do the opposite on when bulking)

- Daily carb intake in calories = 2,358 - 656 - 707 = 995 calories from carbs

- Daily carb intake in grams = 995 / 4 = 248 grams of carbohydrates per day (rounded down from 248.75 grams to prevent eating extra calories)

So, Fred will look to consume 164 grams of protein, 78 grams of fat, and 248 grams of carbohydrates daily for optimal muscle building and fat loss.

If he eats three meals a day and would like to split up his macronutrient intake evenly among his meals for simplicity, at each meal he will eat:

- 54 to 55 grams of protein.

- 26 grams of fat.

- 82 to 83 grams of carbs.

Step #3: Determine Meal Plan Structure

Since Fred works out in the afternoon and his only meal-timing consideration that matters is that he take in 30 to 40 grams of protein within 2 hours before his workout and 30 to 40 grams of protein within 2 hours after his workout, his schedule might look like this:

Meal 1: Pre-workout/late breakfast
Workout
Meal 2: Post-workout/late lunch
Meal 3: Dinner

Alternatively, he could spread out his meals like this:

Meal 1: Breakfast
Meal 2: Pre-workout/lunch
Workout
Meal 3: Post-workout/dinner

Fred's macronutrient profile for each meal is 54 to 55 grams of protein, 26 grams of fat, and 82 to 83 grams of carbs.

So, since a single serving of a protein source is 7 grams of protein, he will need about eight servings of protein per meal.

Carbohydrates will differ based on the type of carbohydrate, so he'll eat different numbers of servings based on the source of the carbs.

A single serving of dietary fat is 5 grams of fat, and the protein servings have some fat, so Fred will need 9 to 15 servings of fat per day. He'll add in his fat sources at the end to round out his diet and create meals.

Knowing about how much of each food source he'll need, Fred can plot out a simple meal layout in his head before determining exactly what to eat and how much.

◇◇◇

There you have it, a full meal plan created from scratch! You can and should follow these exact same steps to create your first meal plan. Once you make your first meal plan and understand how the process works, creating future meal plans becomes easier and easier.

Then adjust as needed only when your weight changes by going back to step #1 above and reworking your calculations.

However, you do have to make the first plan, but as you can see, it's not nearly as difficult as it's made out to be.

CHAPTER 30

HOW TO GET STARTED CORRECTLY

Now that you've done all the calculations, figured out how many calories you should be eating for a perfect cut or bulk, pinned down how much of each macronutrient to eat, and determined what foods and how many servings of each food you'll have for each meal, the real fun begins.

Getting started is always the most difficult, and important, part of any new process. Like trying to push an out-of-gas car down the road, it takes a lot more effort to get started than it does to keep going.

The key is to take those first steps. No matter how bad you think your meal plan is or how many times you've failed in the past, getting started is the most important thing.

Your meal plan and diet are not a burden that you are handcuffed to forever. They form an ever-changing and -improving framework that you can adjust to fit your needs, wants, and cravings.

You now have all the know-how to create a meal plan that is healthy, results-driven, and enjoyable. This meal plan is flexible yet structured, so you can follow it on autopilot and not stress about little hiccups or giving in to your cravings if they should arise.

However, no matter how perfect a meal plan is at the start, it is worthless if you don't follow it and keep improving it. So, you need to consistently keep up with this plan in order to see results.

Staying consistent and tracking your progress are prerequisites for meeting your dietary goals just as they are for reaching your weight-lifting goals. Changing your weight and building more muscle are both long-term processes that require you to know what's working and, more importantly, what isn't working.

This is often where people think about all the work they have to do, get worried, and give up on their diet before they even attempt it. But it shouldn't be.

This is the fun part! Now is the time when you get to reap the fruits of your labor.

As you fulfill your calorie and nutrient needs, your body composition will change. I'm talking about real, noticeable changes to your body in the mirror, on the scale, and in the gym.

It's like a science experiment—add a little more protein here, eat a little bit later in the day there, switch out an apple for raspberries here, try a steak-and-potato recipe there. Each little tweak, week after week, mixes with the others to form this beautiful Frankensteinian monster.

Very few things in life allow you to see the exact changes that are taking place because of your hard work. It truly is an amazing process that picks up speed as you progress.

You start saying no to things, not because you feel you need to have strong willpower, but because you truly don't want, need, or crave them. They're not part of your enjoyable plan.

To make the long-term commitment to this plan easier, the best thing you can do is make it a lifestyle. Eating healthy, much like training, is not a side hobby, a necessary evil, a burden, or an exception. It is the lifestyle you are choosing because you know it will make you feel, look, and function better.

Once you see healthy eating as a nonnegotiable part of a healthy lifestyle, you'll be able to form better and more sustainable habits. It will become almost second nature.

This is why a meal plan is so important. Free-handing your healthy eating will not work, at least not in the beginning.

You may get to a point where you are so aware of what and how much you eat that you won't need to measure anything, but let that be later on. Just stick to your meal plan and make your adjustments along the way. Work foods you enjoy into your plan so adhering to your diet doesn't feel like a Herculean task.

You also don't need to be a food masochist by cutting back on calories today to punish yourself for going over the calorie limit yesterday. Progress is measured in the long term, so long-term consistency, not drastic overcorrection, is the important thing.

If you are feeling like you are either depriving yourself or forcing yourself to eat beyond your limit, that's a sign that something in your meal plan needs to be changed.

Most importantly, diet failure is not a life sentence; it's a learning opportunity. It simply means that your diet is failing you and needs to be adjusted to avoid diet detours in the future.

Constant little improvements week after week will keep you getting results forever.

THE FIRST TWO WEEKS

What gets measured gets improved. If you know exactly what you're putting in your body, including its calories and macronutrients, you will always know whether you are in a calorie deficit or surplus, and you'll be able to adjust accordingly.

Keeping tabs on what you eat and the results you get will keep you on track, help you concentrate on your goals, and allow you to make minor adjustments to get even better results.

Too many people try to jump into a new diet program without ever truly understanding what's in the food they eat and how many calories and macronutrients they are actually eating. One of the major reasons people believe they can't ever be skinny, that they're genetically predisposed to being overweight, or that calorie counting doesn't work is because they have a deep misunderstanding of how many calories they're taking in.

Most people are unable to accurately determine a serving size, the number of calories in a food or meal, or how to properly measure food intake. The vast variety of different foods, companies, and products makes things even more difficult. Worst off are the people who think they are gauging their intake properly and don't understand why they aren't getting the results they believe they should be getting. I believe that's the definition of insanity.

So, to set yourself up for diet success now and in the future, you need to measure and track everything as precisely as possible for the first two weeks—your weight, each food's exact calorie, protein, carbohydrate, and fat content, and how you feel mentally and physically.

As you'll see, tracking your food intake isn't nearly as difficult as people make it out to be. Some people love tracking everything they eat because it provides structure and clarity, while others simply see it as a necessary evil for long-term success. Either way, you only have to track and measure everything for two weeks. Two weeks of tracking provides a good representation of your average schedule, whereas only one week simply isn't long enough for you to get the hang of looking at a serving of food and arriving at a close estimate of its calories and nutrients.

What You Need to Get Started

You should have already completed some of the necessary steps in the previous chapters. You should have:

- A basic meal plan so you can adjust your foods and their servings to better suit your goals. If you simply start measuring everything you're currently eating, all you'll know is how poor your current diet is.

- The stats on your current body weight and physique to help you determine whether your diet is accurate and your body composition is heading in the right direction.

Also, you will need to purchase a few pieces of dieting equipment to accurately and easily track how much you're eating:

- A **digital food scale** to ensure that your food servings are accurate. You can find inexpensive ones on Amazon or at most grocery stores.

- **Food and liquid measuring cups** and utensils for less-accurate but faster measurements.

- A **food tracking sheet or app** for efficient calorie and macronutrient tracking. I recommend a basic notepad or notepad app, a spreadsheet, MyFitnessPal, CalorieKing, or something similar.

The Most Common Reason Calorie Counting Doesn't Work

The recipe you are about to make calls for 320 calories of rice. You pull out your bag of rice and a measuring cup. The nutrition facts panel on your bag of rice says that a half cup, or 87 grams, of rice is 320 calories. So, you pour yourself a half cup of rice, filled to the line, and log 320 calories.

Only, you actually poured yourself 100 grams and 370 calories instead. It's no big deal; it's only 50 calories.

Earlier in the day, you sliced up a medium-size avocado for your sandwich for lunch. Your My-FitnessPal app says a medium-size avocado weighs 136 grams and has 250 calories. So, you log it and move on.

Except the avocado you ate was actually a little larger than "medium-size" and contained 320 calories.

You then repeat this same mistake when measuring a tablespoon of extra virgin olive oil at dinner, the heaping scoop of sugar in your morning coffee, and the steak you weighed *after* cooking it for dinner.

At the end of the day, your calorie deficit has been erased, all due to a bunch of minor mismeasures adding up throughout the day. Simple human errors that you can now use as a learning experience. Instead, here's what you need to do.

How to Accurately Track What You Eat

First, measure the weight of all your food in grams using a food scale. Weighing your foods rather than measuring their volume is more precise and consistent. Do not, I repeat, do NOT worry about trying to get the weight exactly right. You just need to be relatively close.

Second, weigh all your food uncooked. Foods have different water content before and after cooking. Foods like rice or dried pasta will retain water and weigh more after cooking. In contrast, something like a steak will lose moisture and weigh less (it will probably lose some fat too, but don't worry about that). The longer you cook it, the more moisture it will lose, but it will still contain the same nutrition profile.

Third, use products' nutrition facts labels and the USDA database of food nutrients, which you can find on Google. Do it all manually, not just by searching for it in the food tracking apps.

Food tracking apps are notoriously inaccurate, even by as much as a couple of hundred calories a day. Most of their nutrition information comes from user inputs, not actual product nutrition labels.

Fourth, track everything you eat or drink. You must record what you consume, how much you consume, and the total calorie, protein, carbohydrate, and fat content. It's also beneficial to make note of the fiber content in each food. If you add sugar to your coffee, measure how much sugar you use and mark it down. If you put olive oil in a pan before cooking, measure how much oil you use and mark it down. If you're going to eat a handful of chips, weigh them first and mark it down.

This is a lot of work, but you will soon see just how much you eat, the standard calories and nutrients in your most common foods, and how much a specific serving is.

If you learn how to accurately track your calories and macronutrients, you will forever be able to make changes in your body. You don't need to keep up the tracking forever, but if you do hit a plateau or want to minimize errors, you can return to measuring and tracking your food and drinks for a few days to get back on track.

◇◇◇

You now have all the raw knowledge you need on what makes a good diet or meal plan, and how to build one with your specific measurements and goals in mind. And you have the comfort of knowing that dieting does not need to be a long and arduous journey of suffering; it can adapt to your lifestyle, wants, and needs.

That doesn't mean you can eat absolutely anything you want, but still, it's far more flexible than restrictive dieting.

This kind of eating is a major step toward healthy living, and when you know that it is good for you, you're far more likely to want to build a routine and be consistent.

Getting your nutrition right is fundamental to building muscle and having your perfect physique, so don't cut corners or neglect it.

If you're able to nail down creating a meal plan and tracking your food intake, then dieting has just become much easier. You can now slowly work backward from the hard work of getting your out-of-gas car rolling to doing just enough work to keep it moving and coast to your final destination.

We'll discuss how to do this and more in the next part of this book, on progressing and improving.

PART VI

THE PROGRESSION

SECRET 10

–

HOW TO CONSISTENTLY GET
THE BEST POSSIBLE RESULTS

CHAPTER 31

STARTING YOUR BODY-RECOMPOSITION MOMENTUM

In any endeavor, the best way to prevent failure is to plan for it and to completely avoid making little mistakes before they start.

Similarly, the best way to keep building a better and more aesthetic physique is to check that you're applying the basics correctly and that you aren't accidentally overlooking something simple.

Momentum is an amazing force. You can use it in your favor to completely change your body's composition or let it pick up speed in the opposite direction.

Once you start making little mistakes, like getting off your schedule, letting your diet slip, or freestyling your training program, it is much harder to get back on track. Eventually, if you let the little things get away from you, you will hit a plateau or even regress, which can be devastating.

What most people don't realize is that the solution isn't some magical thing they haven't discovered yet. Instead, it's often just a matter of getting back to following the science and the pillars of muscle building and fat loss.

Building muscle and losing fat is a balancing act in which doing too much or too little of one thing can throw off the whole balance and cause you to get poor results.

As someone who struggled for a long time, I know from personal experience how important it is to realize that boring science will always win over promising fitness hacks. It's important to determine what part of the scale is tipping too far in one direction or the other, and what to adjust to balance everything out to return to steadily slimming down, building muscle, and increasing your strength.

As you go through the rest of this chapter, either use it as a checklist to give you confidence that you're doing everything correctly, or use it to understand what you might have overlooked and what you need to adjust to set yourself up for better progression methods in upcoming chapters.

START WITH A BIRD'S-EYE VIEW

Always start by taking a quick bird's-eye view of what is proven to get results, so you don't need to go through every little detail of your programs.

When "recomping," or changing your body's composition, the goal is to change your muscle mass and fat mass at the same time. This requires the fundamental scientific pillars of weight change and muscle building to work together, using a proper diet and strength training as the tools for applying them.

To recomp, you need to eat the correct number of calories based on the number of calories you are expending, i.e., calories in versus calories out, and do it over the long term with a sustainable diet.

You also need to improve how your body partitions and uses nutrients. You do this by building muscle, losing body fat, and improving your health.

The best way to get all three benefits is to eat the correct macronutrients and micronutrients and to strength train. Thus begins the recomping versus just adjusting your weight.

If you strength train to provide high and prolonged tension on your muscles while minimizing metabolic stress and muscle damage, and if you consume the correct macronutrients, number of calories, and water, your body will have the proper stimulus and building blocks to build muscle. As we just touched on, this will also improve your nutrient partitioning.

If you want to keep building muscle, you need to progressively overload your muscles by increasing the intensity or duration of tension that they receive. And you need to allow enough time and provide a good environment for recovery and muscle building to occur.

As you can see, everything intermingles to create body-recomposition momentum. Look at each of the pillars and ensure that you have applied that scientific knowledge.

CHECK YOUR BODY-MEASURING ACCURACY

To be able to make progress toward an amazing body, you need to take measurements and track changes. You shouldn't adjust your programs unless you know that they are definitely failing to deliver on fat loss and muscle building, or are causing issues with your mental or physical health.

Make sure you are following the measuring and tracking basics below.

- Keep notes on how you objectively feel that your training, dieting, health, and well-being are improving.

- Make sure you're tracking body changes over the long term. Your body doesn't change fast enough to make improvements evident from one day to the next.

- Note whether you are getting stronger on your lifts.

- Using a purely subjective approach, check how you appear visually in the mirror.

- Weigh yourself once weekly, first thing in the morning, after going to the bathroom and before drinking or eating anything.

- After weighing yourself, take physique photos in the same environment as you did the previous week.

CHECK FOR POSSIBLE ENERGY BALANCE INACCURACIES

If you have made sure that you are measuring and tracking correctly, the second thing you should do is take a deep look at your nutrition program.

As you know by now, fat loss will mostly come down to the number of calories that you eat or drink compared to the number of calories your body burns in a day. Use the list below to check that you have applied everything correctly.

- Check for and minimize the possibility of overconsuming calories.

- Check that you are not burning fewer calories than you have accounted for.

- Start by making sure your daily calorie intake calculations are correct, i.e., your TDEE and optimal cutting or bulking calories.

- Most people will naturally overestimate their true activity level during the week, so be aware of this and possibly use a lower activity factor.

- The equations assume you have a decent diet and are therefore burning a certain number of calories during digestion (TEF). Try to eat a good amount of whole foods in mixed meals, including fruits and vegetables, fiber, complete proteins, unsaturated fatty acids, and omega-3 fatty acids.

- Finally, make sure you're providing your body with the best potential for building muscles and improving your nutrient partitioning.

OPTIMIZE YOUR MUSCLE-BUILDING POTENTIAL

You want to consistently improve how well your body is able to break down food into nutrients and their substrates, then use the substrates for building muscle rather than fighting important health issues.

Be cognizant of the factors below, which can affect how your body processes nutrients and, in turn, affect your muscle building, fat loss, health, and ability to get results.

- Be certain that you are working to establish a healthy sleep routine to get enough high-quality sleep each night.

- Make adjustments to your daily and weekly routines by training and eating at similar times each day so you can establish a natural biorhythm.

- Be certain that you're using your routine to create habits that help you reduce your stress levels and place your life on autopilot.

- If you haven't already, work to include healthier foods in your diet to improve your health markers and muscle-building potential.

- Prioritize cutting to around 12% body fat to improve how your body processes nutrients and provide your body with optimal muscle-building potential.

- If your health and body fat mass are in check, look at your training program and diet to be certain that you're working toward increasing your muscle mass and strength.

CHECK YOUR TRAINING FACTORS

If your nutrition and lifestyle are on track, then you should take a look at your strength-training program and how you are training. This will come down to making sure your intensity, volume, training frequency, technique, and weight-lifting exercises are dialed in. Here are some specifics to be aware of.

- Be certain that you're using heavy enough weights that you're within 1 rep of technical failure when you reach your desired reps.

- Check that your training experience matches your current set volume. If you are struggling to make progress, you might need to increase or decrease your total sets per muscle.

- Be certain that you are going to the gym motivated to push yourself, conquer your own limitations, and build your dream body.

- Take a look at your technique and be certain that you are doing each exercise correctly.

- Make sure you're performing each exercise with a full range of motion, controlled movements, and both active and passive muscle actions.

244 - **PHYSIQUE SECRETS**

- If you have added exercises to your training program, you may need to return to the basics and decrease the exercise variety.

- Adjust the order of exercises to prioritize what you want to increase strength in and the muscles that need more development.

- Progressively overload your muscles and implement microloading if everything else is taken care of.

IMPLEMENT BETTER PROGRESSION METHODS

So far, everything we've discussed has provided the correct environment to allow you to get results while avoiding minor mistakes that might slow your progress. Building more and more muscle mass, steadily increasing your strength, and slimming down should happen naturally as a result of training and eating correctly.

However, we don't want to just let things happen naturally. We want to provide a catalyst to keep the body-recomposition momentum accelerating. This requires using more advanced strength-training progression methods and applying more program variables.

But to make progress on a diet, you need to be able to change your meal plan quickly and start tracking your food less and less.

In the next two chapters of this section, you'll learn how to use progressive overload, which is the second pillar of building muscle, and sustainability, which is the fourth pillar of modifying your body weight. If you can implement what we cover in the next two chapters, you'll be able to create a truly amazing physique with much less effort.

CHAPTER 32

OPTIMIZING YOUR TRAINING PROGRAM FOR CONSISTENT STRENGTH AND MUSCLE GAINS

Getting stronger and building muscle will happen naturally if you follow the optimal volume, intensity, and frequency recommended in this book. However, it won't be as efficient as it could be, and you will eventually reach an early plateau.

This is the sacrifice you make for simplicity. Unfortunately, it's a necessary sacrifice if you can't stay consistent with your program and lifting technique, or if you don't know how to change the weights to get the right number of reps.

But if you are willing and able to track the weights you use and improve your recovery factors, you should implement the progression strategies we'll discuss in this chapter.

Previously, you could get away with being "close enough" with the weight you used on an exercise or the number of repetitions you performed. The weight you used in one session could have been much heavier or lighter than the previous or the next.

You weren't giving your muscles the exact amount of stress they needed every single training session so that they could maximize strength and growth. This meant you were leaving results on the table.

In this chapter, we'll add the training variables that help you use progressive overload correctly. This way, you can be sure that your training program is working and that you can keep getting stronger and building muscle.

To finish, we'll touch on adjusting your programs when you get injured. Minor injuries and pain are common, so it's important that you know how to work around them to keep making progress.

THE MAIN COMPONENTS

Microloading and deloading, which we talked about in the section on training variables, are the most important parts of progression and proper progressive overload. In this process, you track your training weights and reps and make adjustments to your program as needed. Tracking the weight you used in a session and the number of reps you hit can help you prevent stagnation and be certain you're using the correct weight and reps in the next session.

Also, you should have a structured approach to training and recovery. This means applying the last few training variables so you can provide a consistent and optimal training environment every single session.

It also means that you should try to keep up a good routine and way of life to help your recovery. In this case, we're talking about how well you sleep, how stressed you are, how well you can stick to a training schedule, and whether you have a decent diet.

You don't want to be stuck in a cycle of adding and subtracting weight every other training session because the only time that you put in effort and work hard is an hour a day at the gym.

Tracking Your Weights

You don't want all your hard work to go to waste because you didn't know how to use microloading and deloading correctly. This is especially true if you put in the time to figure out the right volume, intensity, and frequency, as well as which specific exercises will build strength and muscle where you want or need it.

Above all, to avoid wasting time once you set foot in the gym or wherever you're working out, make sure your training program is your best friend. Set it up and follow it diligently.

To ensure that you don't make a mistake or let your memory and ego get in the way, you need to take a completely analytical approach. To do this, it's very important to track your training weights and reps completed and then make the necessary adjustments.

Use a notepad, a printed workout program, a notes app, or a fitness tracker app that allows you to track your weights and reps over at least a few training sessions.

You should write down or make a note of the weight you used for each set and the number of repetitions you completed in each set. While you only really care about the reps on your first set, marking down each set's reps keeps you focused.

Then, before your next training session starts, mark down the amount of weight you will use for each exercise in the next session. You can do this by simply writing down "+2.5 pounds" or "+1 rep" for each exercise.

It's impossible to predict how quickly you will gain strength or recover, but by planning your microloading, you will be aware of it and actively work toward hitting the new weight and reps. Plus, you won't be floundering around the weight section during your workout trying to figure out which weight you should try next.

When tracking your weights, be certain to implement microloading if you hit the reps on the first set. If you missed the mark, be certain to deload and mark down that you need to drop back to a previous training weight in the next session.

You should increase the weight only when you're truly able to complete the required number of repetitions with perfect technique.

Progressive overload is one of the easiest ways to see if you're achieving your goals, but only if you have the correct form and a full range of motion. The temptation to increase a weight and create a false sense of progress may be strong, but you'll only be shooting yourself in the foot.

The Last Few Variables

If you have the correct intensity, the proper number of sets based on your current training level, the right frequency for training each muscle, a core group of exercises that allow you to provide tension on all or most of your muscles, and an effective approach to progressively overloading your muscles, you will see amazing results.

In fact, if you are still progressing in the weight you're lifting and are getting stronger in your current lifts, there is very little reason to make any adjustments to your program. Often, adding in more training variables to concentrate on or adjusting exercises will just throw off the balance of the program and detract from your results.

However, if you are able to stick to a program, are tracking everything, are progressing properly, and have either reached a plateau or become advanced enough to handle more variables, it's time to start optimizing your rest periods, rep tempo, and warm-up.

You should be able to train almost on autopilot and breeze through each training session with minimal thinking about what to do next or how to do it. This means you're able to put all your effort into each exercise, set, and rep. You are completely focused on the weight you're lifting and are pushing yourself to train as hard as you can.

Since you won't have to focus on every little detail that beginners have to actively concentrate on, you have free mental space to begin to time your rest periods, adjust your warm-up so it's perfect for you, and be more cognizant of how fast you're moving the weight you're lifting.

You should be advanced enough that these refinements help you lift more weight and make more consistent gains.

Progressive overload should be used as a gauge to see if you are improving and if your program is working. You can't accurately measure improvement if you have varying warm-up times and intensities, you rest longer between random sets because you're scared that you won't hit the correct reps, or your rep speed is all over the place.

By using each training variable correctly and staying consistent with them, you'll be able to make better progress and know when it's time to implement changes to your program, routine, diet, or lifestyle.

ADJUSTING FOR INJURIES

Having an injury, whether it's from a previous athletic activity, improper strength training, or basic wear and tear, is common.

You should always have your injury evaluated by a medical professional and make sure you're cleared before you get back into training. Once you are cleared, it can be beneficial to adjust the amount, intensity, and exercise choice in order to keep building muscle while preventing exacerbation of the injury.

Unfortunately, most people stop working out when they sustain an injury. In fact, many see injuries as an excuse for not exercising. However, exercise significantly speeds up the recovery process.

In other words, exercise can be used as a treatment for injuries. It accelerates the healing process. Doctors wouldn't often prescribe physiotherapy to injured people if all exercise worsened injuries.

Studies also indicate that active recovery speeds up tissue repair.[1] That is, of course, if it is done correctly.

So, instead of quitting following an injury or discomfort beyond normal fatigue, I recommend that you modify your training program to make it sustainable. Here are the steps you should follow, in order:

1. First, reduce the possibility of exacerbating the injury without changing your program.

   a. Allow enough rest time between sets. Increase your rest periods to ensure that your muscles, tendons, joints, and neuromuscular system are recovered and won't be overly fatigued.
   b. Drop back on your proximity to failure while focusing on proper technique. If you are staying only 1 rep away from failure, you should increase this to 2 or 3 reps.
   c. Lower your repetition speed. Slow down how fast you move the weight to ensure proper technique and prevent extra stress.

4. Adjust the amount of stress placed on your muscles, joints, ligaments, etc., at a given time, i.e., your training intensity. Do this by reducing the weight you use. Instead of putting more stress on the injury by trying to lift very heavy weights, decrease the amount of weight and increase the number of reps. You can go all the way up to 20 to 30 reps if needed.

5. Reduce the total amount of stress per week and per training session, i.e., your training volume, by lowering the total number of sets per week. You might be doing too much volume, which is causing you pain and creating injuries. This is often a sign of overtraining, which is a nightmare for recovery and healing. Cut back on the number of sets per week by 2 or 3 or more for the injured muscle. Reducing volume (sets per muscle per week) is beneficial only for an overtrained muscle or ligament.

6. Adjust your entire training program schedule or format. Changing your entire program is much more difficult than most people realize. Little mistakes, like failing to account for adjusted training volume per muscle with an alternative exercise, can ruin muscle and strength development.

a. Replace exercises that cause pain with one or more exercises that stress the same muscles but don't cause pain. This could mean switching from a barbell to dumbbells or cables. You can also adjust your grip and grip width. Here are two common examples:

   i. Due to improper technique and overtraining of the pecs, shoulder pain and discomfort during the barbell bench press is common. Switching to dumbbells (assuming you use proper technique) or a narrow grip with elbows tucked to your sides can often alleviate discomfort. Swapping the flat bench press for an incline variation can also reduce discomfort for some people.

   ii. Knee, hip, or lower back pain is common, especially when squatting. This is often due to prior injuries, poor technique, or a lagging muscle group, such as a weak lower back compared to the quads. If you're unable to do exercises like the Bulgarian split squat or reverse lunge due to pain with spinal loading exercises, a machine leg press might be necessary. To ensure that your training volume per muscle stays consistent, you'd need to replace a back squat with both a leg press variation and a back hyperextension variation. You might also need to add a couple of sets of planks to your program to account for the reduced transverse abdominis development owing to a flexed midsection throughout the back squat.

c. Reduce your training frequency. This should be a last resort, but instead of training a muscle about every 3½ days, you can increase the time in between to 5 to 7 days to allow a longer recovery period between sessions.

CHAPTER 33

HOW TO GET A LIFETIME OF CONSISTENT RESULTS FROM YOUR DIET

Hopefully by now I've burned this into your brain, but building muscle and strength and leaning out is a long-term process that ideally becomes a complete lifestyle change.

This requires consistency, as we have also discussed many times. You need to consistently eat the correct quality and quantity of foods in the long term in order to see results.

You can change up what you eat and experiment with new things, or be a bit indulgent every now and again at a family dinner, but the bulk of your nutrition should be planned and prepared for the best results.

Just as importantly, you need to keep adjusting your program based on the results you are getting. This requires a decent amount of tracking of your food, body weight, and body composition, which should also become routine.

However, tracking your food intake and its calories and macronutrients is very rarely sustainable for people who aren't actively trying to get to single-digit body fat levels or who are not in the fitness and nutrition industries.

In fact, for most people, real success comes when you're able to get results with as minimal tracking as possible while also being able to adjust your meal plan to match your changing body weight and composition. This requires a transition from the first two weeks of a diet plan, when maximal accuracy and tracking are required to establish proper eating habits, gain experience with tracking and measuring, and allow your body to respond and adjust to your new diet.

I always suggest that people stick to any new meal plan for a week or two before revising it. Your body takes time to respond and adjust, so about two weeks will give you enough time to gauge any changes that your body is going through.

After a week or two of your meal plan, adjust it if necessary for your new measurements and weight. Finding a balance is important, as you don't want to obsess over your body weight, but you do need to be cognizant of it.

As you begin to work out and eat according to your training and nutrition plan, your body will build muscle and lose fat. After a few weeks, your body weight and composition will change. You will have progressed both physically and knowledge-wise. You will have learned the types of foods to eat, how to track your food, how to calculate your calories accurately and easily, how to time your meals, and much more.

As you progress, you will need to adjust your nutrition plan based on this progress to keep getting the best results possible.

In the same way, you should slowly move toward a tracking target that you can always hit. As we discussed in the previous section, you should track your food intake based on the results versus the flexibility you want.

To do this properly, you will need to work backward from purely external measuring methods, like a food scale, to internal measuring methods, like hunger.

By aiming for the right tracking target combined with adjusting your meal plan as your body changes, you'll be able to get sustainable results for life.

HOW TO QUICKLY ADJUST YOUR MEAL PLAN FOR CONTINUAL IMPROVEMENT

You can quickly adapt your nutrition program by adjusting your meal plan either weekly or every other week based on your weight change, or by maintaining the same meal plan until you hit a plateau.

Option #1: Adjusting Weekly or Every Other Week

I suggest weighing yourself each week and adjusting your daily calorie intake in accordance with your weight changes. This will allow you to prepare meals, plan for the week, be certain that your diet is working, and stay focused on your goals.

Adjusting your diet should be simple and quick. If you like your diet's current structure, then you have a few options for adjusting your calories and macronutrients without needing to restart each week.

Your first option is to slightly shrink the serving sizes of all your meals or of a single meal or macronutrient. For example, you can take 5 grams of carbs, 3 grams of fat, and 3 grams of protein off each meal. If you eat three meals a day, this would be about 177 calories a day.

Another approach to this option is to maintain your protein and fat intakes but lower your carbohydrate intake by 25 to 50 grams over the whole day. This would be 100 to 200 calories a day and can easily be done without retooling much of your diet.

Your second option is to replace calorie-dense foods with nutrient-dense foods or choose lower-calorie versions of similar, higher-calorie products. For example, try substituting low-calorie sweeteners for table sugar, using low-fat and low-sugar varieties of certain foods, eating fresh fruit instead of a gummy fruit snack, or eating a whole piece of fruit rather than drinking it or getting it out of a can.

Just make consistent, slight adjustments. These will add up over time without requiring big sacrifices.

Option #2: Adjusting Based on Plateaus

If you don't want to keep weighing yourself and slightly adjusting your meal plan and are willing to sacrifice results, you can stick to your current diet until you hit a plateau and then recalculate.

Here's what I mean: Suppose you weighed 220 pounds (about 100 kilograms) before beginning your diet plan. After a number of weeks, you weigh 190 pounds, but you've hit a plateau. You are staying loyal to your eating plan and working hard, but you can't lose weight anymore. When this happens, you'll need to recalculate to make sure the number of calories you eat every day is right for your weight.

Remember, the first calculation you made on calorie adjustment was for a 220-pound person, not for a 190-pound person. So, the fat-loss plan you created for a 220-pound person has now become a maintenance plan for a 190-pound person.

Time to readjust your eating plan. In other words, you need to recalculate your daily calorie intake based on your new weight, which in this example is 190 pounds.

Follow the new plan until you reach a plateau again and recalculate. Repeat this until you get the results you want.

MOVING FORWARD BY WORKING BACKWARD

To be able to transition from having complete accuracy but only short-term consistency, such as in the first two weeks of a diet plan, you need to work backward.

To get the best accuracy with your meal plan and, in turn, the best results, your measuring and tracking in the initial weeks should have primarily come from physical tracking methods that involved actual, quantifiable measurements. These are weighing your food, tracking your own weight, measuring your body composition, and noticing when your performance improves.

But to guide your diet throughout the year, you should look to establish proper eating habits and rely on your body's internal cues, like feelings of hunger, fullness, and well-being. Then, when the results you're getting run counter to the direction your internal cues are leading you, you can start tracking to reestablish better habits, get back on track, or break through a plateau.

Implementing a Backwards Approach

The goal in dieting is to get to the best body composition that you can healthily maintain. You need a sustainable approach to eating if this is ever going to happen.

This starts with first having experience dieting to build muscle and lose fat. It involves creating a meal plan, maintaining an eating structure, adjusting serving sizes, tracking your food, and understanding which foods to eat for health and satiety.

If you don't know what you're doing, you won't know why you aren't getting results.

To implement a backwards approach to dieting, here are your steps:

1. Start by aiming for the farthest tracking target: track everything and establish good diet awareness.

2. When ready, aim for the middle target: reduce tracking to only protein and calories.

3. If your body composition is still progressing properly, move to the closest target and concentrate mostly on your own hunger to guide you: reduce to tracking only protein or only calories, depending on your diet awareness and goals.

4. Maintain this until your body composition stops changing the way you want it to. Then increase your servings of healthy and satiating foods or go back to tracking calories and protein again.

You can follow these rules for as long as you need to and combine them with the food tracking guidelines discussed in chapter 30.

After a month or two of trial and error, you should be able to listen to your body's hunger and satiety cues to help you determine whether you're eating too much or too little, or whether your body fat is too high or too low.

SECRET 11

-

TIPPING THE SCALES

CHAPTER 34

THE SMALL THINGS
THAT CAN HELP GIVE
A FINAL PUSH

There is a reason that this section is at the very end of *Physique Secrets*. Tipping a scale, nonmeta-phorically, takes only a tiny amount of weight added to one side to get that side to be heavier and "tip."

The biggest results will come from everything we have put on the scale leading up to this.

Your top priorities should always be to slowly implement each of the different training variables, keep track of your training weights, measure your progress, and build a solid routine that optimizes your recovery factors and puts your training and nutrition on autopilot.

Likewise with your diet, it's crucial to have a structured, balanced, and flexible meal plan, track your calorie and macronutrient intakes, measure your progress, implement any needed changes to your plan, and make sure it is enjoyable and sustainable. Mastering these tactics will bring you success not just now but for the rest of your life.

When you make both strength training and nutrition integral parts of your lifestyle rather than necessary evils, creating the body you want becomes an enjoyable process, not a chore.

If you can do all of that correctly, I guarantee that you will build an amazing physique.

Still, there may come a time when you want, or need, to tip the scales on your fat loss or muscle building. You might have reached a strength or muscle-building plateau and need just a slight push to keep improving. Maybe you are at a single-digit body fat percentage, are having trouble cutting any more calories from your diet, and would like a way to burn a few extra calories without making any substantial changes. Or maybe you just want to get in better cardiovascular shape, or you have supplement money burning a hole in your pocket.

As you can probably tell, tipping the scales is about adopting that last little bit of programming to break through plateaus or gain a slight edge. This means that you should do cardio and take supplements at certain times and for certain reasons.

WHEN TO ADD CARDIO TO YOUR TRAINING PROGRAM

You do not need cardio to build a lean and amazing body. In fact, most of the time, you should avoid doing cardio and instead pour your effort into strength training and perfecting your diet.

Personally, I have little trouble getting down to 7%–8% body fat without doing more than 10 minutes of light cardio as a warm-up. If I ever had the desire to drop below 7%–8%, I might add in as little cardio as needed strictly for fat loss.

Plus, by avoiding doing cardio, except during a warm-up, I tend to spend less time in the gym, am able to lift more intensely during my workout, and have more energy even when performing a cut.

However, you don't need to avoid cardio like the plague, because it does offer some benefits when done correctly by certain people.

In general, you should add cardio to your program only when (1) you want or need to build better cardiovascular endurance or (2) your body fat level is very high or low.

For building better cardiovascular endurance, add in cardio if you:

- Are a complete beginner who needs to form a foundation of fitness.

- Need help with recovery and breathing between sets.

- Do short strength-training sessions.

- Want to add cardio and are willing to sacrifice strength-training results.

When it comes to fat loss specifically, add in cardio if you:

- Are at a very low body fat percentage (8%–9% or less) and need to tip the scales.

- Have a very high body fat percentage (25% or higher) and need to lose weight quickly.

If you don't fit into any of these situations, then you will get better results by limiting the amount of cardio you do, or doing none at all (except for your warm-up).

However, if any of these descriptions do apply to you, in the next chapter we will discuss cardio, its pros and cons for developing an aesthetic physique, and the best methods of performing cardio.

WHEN TO ADD SUPPLEMENTS TO YOUR REGIMEN

Supplements can be broken down into three main categories based on their functions in your body:

- General health

- Muscle building and performance enhancement

- Fat loss or fat burning

General health supplements are designed to fill in any missing nutrients that you might not get from your diet.

Muscle-building and performance-enhancing supplements are designed to provide nutrients to your muscles and help you train harder and recover faster. In the upcoming chapter on supplements, I will not include any anabolic agents.

"Fat-burning" supplements don't actually burn fat but help to increase your metabolism so that you burn a few more calories during the day.

If there were one magic fat-loss or muscle-building supplement that was proven effective with minimal side effects, it wouldn't be sold as a supplement. The pharmaceutical companies would sell it as medicine and jack up the price—look at testosterone and steroids for proof.

To save you time and money, there are NO PROVEN, LEGAL, or SAFE supplements that can make you gain muscle or shed fat from your body without putting in the effort in the gym and kitchen.

That being said, although supplements aren't the holy grail most people desire, they can be used in certain scenarios to help you tip the scales.

Scenario #1: You need to boost your nutrient intake.

To improve your health, you should take a multivitamin and fish oil supplement. You might also benefit from creatine supplementation for your brain and nervous system.

Also, if you struggle with consuming enough protein during the day, you might benefit from adding a mixed protein powder to your supplement regimen.

Scenario #2: You want a slight edge.

If you are following a quality training program and diet, and supplements won't become a substitute for hard work, you can add in all of the supplements I'll recommend later in the book, or pick and choose as you wish.

Scenario #3: You have hit a strength- and muscle-building plateau.

Adding creatine monohydrate, beta-alanine, and caffeine supplements can help increase your muscle-building potential.

Creatine increases the amount of work you can do during your workouts by helping with energy and power for muscle contractions. This means you can do more reps with heavier weights, which leads to more potential for your muscles to grow.

Beta-alanine increases the amount of work you can complete because it helps with muscle buffering and metabolic stress. This can help you do more repetitions in a training session.

And caffeine can raise your energy levels and blunt your perception of fatigue, which, again, helps you accomplish more work during a training session.

Scenario #4: You have hit a fat-loss plateau.

If you have a dialed-in diet and are tracking and measuring properly, and you are at a low body fat percentage, then adding in fish oil, creatine monohydrate, beta-alanine, and caffeine supplements can help augment your fat-loss potential.

Omega-3 fatty acids can directly impact your protein synthesis and fat metabolism rates while also improving many aspects of mental and physical health. To ensure that you get enough omega-3s, supplementation with fish oil is often recommended.

As mentioned above, creatine, beta-alanine, and caffeine all help you train more intensely, complete more work during a training session, and build muscle. Besides improving nutrient partitioning, this causes you to burn more calories (1) while training, (2) through the body's work to produce new muscle mass, and (3) to maintain the increased muscle mass.

Also, caffeine revs up your metabolism by increasing your heart rate. This results in a small but consistent uptick in calories burned daily.

These extra calories burned can be just enough to tip the scales in your fat-loss favor.

CHAPTER 35

CARDIO FOR AESTHETICS

When most people think about exercising for fat loss, they immediately think of cardiovascular (cardio) training—such as running on a treadmill or riding a stationary bike. This conjures up the image of spending many hours on the treadmill, breathing heavily and sweating their butts off to drop a few pounds.

Cardio is important if your major goal is to train your cardiovascular system and you don't feel that strength training is already providing you with these benefits (although it is).

Other than that, whether or not to do cardio seems like a pretty straightforward cost-to-benefit decision.

The cost is how much of your time you're willing to sacrifice in return for the benefit of burning more calories.

This misguided logic is very short-sighted because it overlooks the true cost of doing cardio when it comes to not only losing fat and burning calories, but also developing muscle, staving off hunger, having energy throughout the day, and more.

There are certain times when you can and should do cardio based on the benefits that come with it, and there are specific ways to perform cardio to maximize the benefits while minimizing the negative costs.

In the end, it will be your choice to do cardio or not, but first you need to understand that it's not the fat-loss panacea some "influencers" and coaches believe it is. In fact, adding cardio can often make your physique worse.

CARDIO VERSUS AESTHETICS

As you should know, for fat loss, exercise is not more effective than simply eating equivalently fewer calories, and research has proven diet to be the primary controller of weight loss.[1]

However, when done correctly, exercise can help tip the scales.

You should understand that adding more strength training isn't a viable option for burning more calories. Excessive strength training will result in poorer recovery, overtraining, less muscle development, more fatigue, an increased possibility of injuries, and ultimately less fat loss. In other words, a worse physique.

This is typically why people add cardio to their programs. But cardio is a double-edged sword when it comes to achieving a great physique. It can interfere with your muscle- and strength-gain goals in both the short and the long term.

In the short term, you do burn calories, which can help with fat loss; but excessive cardio bouts can also break down muscle mass. Cardio also increases muscle, neural, and mental fatigue, making it impossible to strength train as hard as you would otherwise, which will decrease the amount of muscle you can build.

The long-term effects of cardio for fat loss make things even worse.

Basically, your body isn't good at adapting to two different things. You can either be really good at endurance activities or be strong and muscular.

When you do both cardio and strength training, a real phenomenon is created called the "interference effect." Cardio disrupts the cell signaling that promotes muscle growth.[2] This hampers your strength training by decreasing your strength and muscle-mass gains.[3]

Many studies have shown that endurance training directly interferes with muscle growth, strength, and power.

A meta-analysis comparing 21 different high-quality studies found that people doing both endurance training and strength training gained only 69% as much muscle as those doing strictly strength training.

In addition, the strength of the endurance-and-strength-training group was 82% of that of the strength-training-only group—which isn't as bad as the muscle-gain difference, but still isn't ideal.[4]

So, if your goal is to have an aesthetic physique, which I'm sure you are here for, then spend your energy strength training and monitoring your calorie intake and keep cardio to a minimum.

HOW TO DO CARDIO FOR OPTIMAL RESULTS

In chapter 34, we discussed the few times that you should do cardio. You might need to flip back to that page to determine whether you fit into any of the categories.

If you do fit into any of those categories, the two types of cardio that I recommend are walking and, at select times, high-intensity interval training (HIIT).

HIIT workouts should only be done by people who are new to working out and strength training, people with higher body fat levels, or people wanting to get into great cardio shape. Outside of those scenarios, avoid HIIT and do low-intensity cardio when you're looking for extra fat loss.

Debunking the HIIT Myth

HIIT cardio has become the flavor of the week and is used as a buzzword to make a workout sound fancy or super-difficult. A lot of trainers promise that with HIIT you will burn extensive amounts of body fat and place your body in a fat-burning state for the next 24 to 48 hours.

In reality, you burn only a measly number of calories more than you would burn normally without an "afterburn" effect.[5] This afterburn is known scientifically as excess post-exercise oxygen consumption, or EPOC, and it lasts only a few minutes to a couple of hours.

In fact, a systematic review of 21 different studies looking at EPOC, low-intensity exercise, moderate-intensity exercise, and high-intensity exercise found that a HIIT session averages only about 50 extra calories burned over a whole day.[6]

HIIT is also hard on the body and is nearly impossible to stick with for even a few training sessions, let alone over the long term, making it a poor training style.

Finally, outside of the novice strength-training stage, HIIT will hinder you from putting on muscle mass because it has a strong interference effect.[7]

The Best Cardio Method for Fat Loss: Low-Intensity Steady-State (LISS) Walking

Research has shown low-intensity steady-state (LISS) cardio to be more effective than HIIT for fat loss.[8]

Walking is one of the easiest low-intensity steady-state cardio exercises you can do. In fact, it doesn't make you feel that you are actually doing cardio. It is a simple and effective way to burn a few extra calories.

Walking workouts could be anything from taking your dogs for a walk, hiking, taking a stroll while talking on the phone, walking to work or the store, walking on a treadmill after weight lifting, or anything else you can think of.

As a goal, you should look to get anywhere from 8,000 to 10,000 steps in a day. But this is not necessary, and the exact number of steps doesn't really matter.

The Best Cardio Method for Novices: High-Intensity Interval Training (HIIT)

HIIT has been shown to help with fat loss while maintaining muscle mass when done correctly and only for select populations, which we discussed.[9]

For HIIT, you work at 90% or more of your maximum effort for a short time, followed by a period of rest or a slower pace. This might sound eerily similar to strength training; it's weird how that works.

But keep in mind, HIIT can be intense and hard on the body, especially if you are doing it on a treadmill or running on concrete, so it's recommended that you do it only three or four times a week and for 10 to 15 minutes, tops.

For HIIT to be effective (for fat loss and muscle maintenance), you need to do it at a 1:4 work-to-rest ratio. This means you need to go all out or close to it for a quarter as long as you rest or go at a much slower pace. And the work period should be 20 seconds at most.

For example, you can do 10-second sprints separated by 40-second rest periods, or do 15-second sprints with 1 minute of slow walking after each. Your mode of cardio is not that important.

A CARDIO SCHEDULE FOR THE FEW WHO WILL BENEFIT

On workout days:

1. 10–15 minutes of walking, biking, or stair stepper for warm-up.

2. Strength-training workout.

3. 10–20 minutes of walking or 5 rounds of 15-second intervals followed by 60 seconds of slow pace, either running, biking, rowing, or stair stepper. Slowly work to increase your speed and intensity, then add time if you are still not seeing results.

On nonworkout days, choose one of the following options:

a. 1 hour of light cardio a day.

b. 10 minutes of HIIT: 10 seconds 90% sprint followed by 40 seconds slow pace or resting. Your choice of cardio method (bike, running, stair stepper, hill climbing, rowing, elliptical, etc.).

You can spread out the cardio throughout your day based on what fits your schedule and preferences. For example, instead of doing a full hour, you could do 20 minutes in the morning, 20 minutes at lunch, and 20 minutes after work.

I made this schedule so you don't have to go to the gym at all on days when you don't lift. Go really hard those days and really easy the rest of the time.

On your rest day, you should completely rest. This is a day completely off from any intensive exercise so that your body recovers and grows.

The goal is to do as little cardio as possible while maximizing your strength training and muscle building.

◇◇◇

As you can see, the cost-to-benefit of doing cardio is a lot more complicated than simply exchanging time and effort for being leaner.

If you want to build more muscle, burn more calories during the day, suppress your appetite, and spend less time and energy working out, you need to put all your effort into strength training. Add light cardio only if you are at a very low body fat percentage, to avoid nutrient deficiencies. Other than that, avoid cardio!

CHAPTER 36

THE FEW SUPPLEMENTS WORTH ADDING TO YOUR REGIMEN

The supplement industry is a multi-billion-dollar industry, and supplement companies' goal is to sell you their products at any cost. If they make a sale, they win; they don't care whether you win or lose.

Each claims its product is the newest and best thing on the market, but which supplements are actually worth their weight, and which are snake oil?

The supplements worth taking satisfy five rules.

Rule #1: They actually do what they say they do.

I will outline the only supplements that have been heavily researched and shown to live up to their claims. If a supplement isn't mentioned, that means it either does not back up the claims or there hasn't been enough research done on it to determine whether it works.

Rule #2: They are safe and healthy to take.

The pros of putting a substance in your body should far outweigh the cons. The supplements I'm going to discuss are the ones that are recommended to professional athletes by sports dietitians due to their good performance and low risk of adverse effects. Each is very safe at the recommended dosage.

Rule #3: They are supplements, not substitutes.

Supplements are supposed to help you get results after you already have a solid eating plan and understand proper nutrition. That's why they're called supplements—they are supplemental to your hard work and good nutrition. They are not a substitute. You should never use a supplement to replace real food or a change in your eating and training.

Rule #4: Their effectiveness is worth the money.

You want to get your money's worth from a supplement. If you're spending $39.99 a month on a supplement that's giving you $8 worth of results, then the supplement isn't worth it.

Rule #5: They come from reputable sources or companies.

When you're deciding on a supplement, make sure the brand you're buying is certified by a third-party laboratory and is free of banned substances and other contaminants. Every batch should be tested and certified for purity.

Numerous prominent supplement companies have been sued for adding ingredients that were not listed on the ingredient label so that people could get a better response to their products.

And of course, a lot of the claims and research touted by supplement companies are misleading and inaccurate. Do your research and don't sacrifice your health for a "shortcut."

With these things in mind, let's zero in on which supplements can help you tip the scales!

I want to make it clear that I have no financial stake in any supplement products. So, I can tell you without bias and based on research what you should spend your money on and what you should stay away from because of marketing hype.

RECOMMENDED SUPPLEMENTS

I recommend only six types of supplements. All are well backed by research, have little to no side effects, are cost effective, and can help you build a better physique.

These six supplements are:

1. Multivitamins

2. Fish oil

3. Caffeine

4. Mixed protein powders

5. Creatine monohydrate

6. Beta-alanine

Let's take a closer look at each of these.

Multivitamins

The research behind multivitamins is a bit inconclusive, since there are so many different manufacturers with different amounts of vitamins and minerals in their products. Nevertheless, multivitamins are recommended by sports dietitians and the American Medical Association for the general population.

This is because some studies have shown that multivitamins can help you get the vitamins and minerals that you may be lacking in your diet.[1] It's better to get your vitamins and minerals from real food, but most of the time, people are not able to take in all of the recommended dosages and vitamins every day. A multivitamin will help fill in the gaps, but it should be used only as an extra, not as a way to allow yourself to eat unhealthy food.

Taking a multivitamin isn't going to help you lift more, run faster, or build muscle, but it will help prevent micronutrient deficiencies that could impair your performance and health.

If you feel that you are deficient in certain vitamins or minerals, it is important to get checked out by a doctor.

Fish Oil

Fish oil is the oil obtained from certain kinds of fish—exactly what it sounds like. It is rich in the omega-3 essential fatty acids, specifically the polyunsaturated fatty acids eicosapentaenoic acid (EPA) and docosahexaenoic acid (DHA).

Our bodies cannot produce omega-3 fatty acids, and yet these nutrients are very important when it comes to our health, muscle growth, and fat loss. Therefore, we must consume omega-3s in our diet.

Most people,though, rarely eat salmon, mackerel, tuna, and other great sources of omega-3s, which makes it difficult to take in the optimal amount of these essential nutrients. As a result, it's a good idea to supplement with fish oil, or an alternative like krill or algae oil, daily for optimal health.

Supplement with 0.5 to 3 grams daily of an omega-3 fatty acid supplement that contains both EPA and DHA, most likely fish oil, from a reputable company.

Still, you should try your best to get omega-3 fatty acids from your meals. Oily fish are high-quality protein sources, and a lot of fish oil supplements are of low quality.[2]

It's vitally important to make sure to find omega-3 supplements that are pure and non-oxidized, as validated by an independent lab. Oxidized omega-3 supplements can be very unsafe, and you don't want to be paying for poison.

Caffeine

Caffeine is one of the most widely used drugs and supplements on the market. It can help increase your workout capacity and ramp up your metabolism to enhance fat loss.

When it comes to enhancing training performance, there are two leading theories explaining caffeine's effectiveness.[3]

First, caffeine is believed to make you perceive that you are doing less work than you really are, which can help you complete more repetitions in a workout before your body or mind fatigues.

Second, it's believed that chemicals caffeine causes to be released from the brain help improve muscle contraction, which, in turn, allows you to lift more weight without realizing you're working harder.[4]

Caffeine has also been shown to help people lose fat by speeding up both heart rate and metabolism. As a result, the body ends up burning more calories throughout the day.[5]

Based on research, the recommended dosage of caffeine is 1.3 to 2.7 milligrams per pound of body weight (or 3 to 6 milligrams per kilogram) about an hour before exercise or during longer exercise bouts. Higher doses do not result in greater performance improvements.[6]

Personally, I believe this dosage is too high for most people, so start at a lower dosage and increase it if needed. Caffeine can have a wide range of side effects, so it's up to you to determine whether your body can handle caffeine ingestion.

Mixed Protein Powders

Protein powders are hugely popular among weight lifters and bodybuilders, many of whom guzzle down protein shakes like they are muscles in a shaker bottle.

But the most reliable and effective way to stimulate protein synthesis and reduce the breakdown of proteins to enhance muscle building is to consume the proteins from whole foods as opposed to processed protein powders. Research has found that whole-food protein sources—whole milk, for example—stimulate more protein balance than processed protein sources like skim milk.[7]

Many whole-food sources of protein are also great sources of vitamins, minerals, and other micronutrients, which are very important for the nutritional quality of your diet and which protein supplements cannot provide.

Eating your calories is also more filling than drinking them. Take, for example, eating 6 ounces of steak versus drinking 12 ounces of water mixed with two scoops of protein powder. Both have about 45 grams of protein, but steak is far more filling.

The only time you should consider adding protein powder to your supplement protocol is if you struggle to consume enough protein in your daily meals due to getting full, not liking the food, being a vegan or vegetarian, or not having enough time to prepare meals.

If you do decide to add protein powders, mixed protein powders are superior to single-sourced protein powders.

Look for a mixed protein powder that has more micellar casein protein than whey protein isolate. Both casein and whey are proteins derived from milk and have their benefits when it comes to speed of digestion, but research has shown that casein does a better job at stimulating cumulative muscle protein synthesis, thus enhancing muscle growth.[8]

Research shows that protein sources with faster absorption speeds, like whey, do not stimulate muscle protein synthesis for as long as slower proteins.[9] This means whey causes a large spike in muscle protein synthesis but less muscle growth over time.

Micellar casein is a slow-digesting protein source that provides a steady flow of amino acids. This helps prevent muscle protein breakdown and improves muscle protein synthesis.

A mixed protein powder containing both micellar casein and whey isolate will offer both fast absorption and a sustained release of amino acids—the best of both worlds. In fact, a mixed powder of 80% casein and only 20% whey protein has been shown to promote protein synthesis the most. This is very close to the protein content of standard whole milk.

If you do not eat or drink milk products, you can use a protein powder made from eggs or beef. Both offer the same benefits (amino acids), but both are typically much more expensive with no extra benefits.

Even more expensive is collagen protein or collagen peptides. These are becoming very popular as a fountain of youth and recovery supplement, but they have no benefit if you consume enough vitamin C and protein. Save your money.

If you are vegan or vegetarian, or you don't consume any animal, milk, or egg proteins, look for a mixed pea and rice protein powder with a ratio of 80:20 pea to rice. These sources offer a complementary amino acid profile, so you avoid the common plant protein problem of not having enough of every amino acid.

Along those lines, soy protein powder has a poor amino acid and bioavailability profile, so it is not worth using.

Creatine Monohydrate

Creatine is one of the most important natural fuel-enhancing components for strength trainers. Creatine, especially creatine monohydrate, has been studied a lot more than most other supplements and has been shown to work and be safe.

Creatine is used inside your muscle fibers to create creatine phosphate and replenish adenosine triphosphate (ATP). Both molecules help provide energy for muscle contraction and short, fast bursts of activity. This helps you complete more work, improve performance, and train harder, which can translate into greater muscle gains.

Research has backed this up by showing that creatine supplementation can help improve your workout capacity, thus enhancing strength development and muscle growth.[10]

It's important to understand that creatine does not create muscle; it allows you to push more intensely in your workouts, which provides the potential for more muscle. That is, if you actually work harder.

To add to the positives of creatine, it can improve the health of your brain and central nervous system.

Creatine monohydrate is the most studied form of creatine, and all other creatine forms have repeatedly paled in comparison. So, creatine monohydrate is the proven gold standard.

Take 3 to 5 grams of creatine monohydrate per day; timing is unimportant. Because your muscles must first increase their creatine stores, it will take two to four weeks before any noticeable effects.

It's important to note that creatine supplements have received some bad press for causing adverse side effects. However, numerous studies have been unable to find any negative side effects from its use when dosage recommendations are followed.

Beta-alanine

Beta-alanine is an amino acid that has become popular in the nutrition market as a way to potentially work out longer and with more intensity before muscle fatigue sets in.

Multiple studies have shown that beta-alanine allows people who are resistance training to complete more repetitions before fatigue, after about three to four weeks of supplementation.[11] This is because beta-alanine combines with histidine in skeletal muscles to create carnosine. Carnosine helps with clearing hydrogen ions from muscle fibers and slowing the onset of metabolic stress.

This is called "muscle buffering," and it is linked to less muscle fatigue and possibly the ability to work out harder, longer. Buffering nutrients out of your muscles and decreasing metabolic stress might allow you to increase the tension you're able to place on your muscles, which will in turn increase the potential for developing muscles.

Research has shown that beta-alanine is the limiting factor for creating carnosine in your muscles, so by increasing the limiting factor, your muscles will be able to create more carnosine. Therefore, beta-alanine has the greatest influence on carnosine levels in your muscles.[12] And there is no advantage to taking carnosine, since it is immediately broken down into beta-alanine and histidine during digestion.

The recommended dosage of beta-alanine is 3 to 6 grams per day, taken as 1.5 to 3 grams twice a day, since beta-alanine can cause flushing and itching of the skin upon ingestion. It takes about four weeks to get the maximum benefits of beta-alanine, because carnosine stores need to build up in your muscles first.

It's important to remember that, like creatine, beta-alanine does not build muscles. It simply allows you to work out harder, which, if supported by proper nutrition, can help you develop muscle and burn more calories.

◇◇◇

Do what you can to get your nutrients from whole foods. Supplements are not as important as people think. In fact, you don't need any supplementation to get an amazing physique.

The goal of the supplement industry is to make money, and manufacturers will do whatever it takes to get money from desperate people. We don't have that much else to sell in the fitness industry, and supplements are easy to produce and profitable.

You shouldn't be surprised that most bodybuilding and fat-loss supplements on the market are flops. You don't need to waste hundreds, or even thousands, of dollars every month on supplements. Most of them are worthless.

However, there are a few that may help tip the scales if you struggle with getting your nutrients from your meals. Stick to the brands that are trustworthy.

THE CONCLUSION

THE END IS JUST
THE BEGINNING

Congratulations! You now have everything you need to get started on your journey to building a phenomenal physique, both inside and out.

In *Physique Secrets*, I've given you scientifically proven information that will supply you with all the tools you need to build muscle and strength while getting rid of unwanted body fat.

My goal was to provide you with a solid foundation on which to build an amazing body. Building on that foundation is yours to see through. All the information in this book will be trivial if you don't put it into action.

Every individual has their own personal preferences and goals when it comes to building an aesthetic physique, so strive for what makes you happy and healthy. Some people see an athletic physique as aesthetically pleasing, others love muscular and huge bodies, while still others prefer a physique with just a little muscle.

The choice of the physique that you want is yours, as long as your body has the genetic potential to achieve it and it doesn't require an unhealthy approach.

Throughout *Physique Secrets*, I've provided you with the most important guidelines and principles for creating a proportionate and symmetrical body that flows from broad shoulders into a nice, tapered V shape.

To get this amazing body, you need to work on developing each of your visible and trainable muscles to its fullest potential while keeping your body fat percentage low enough to show off these muscles. To achieve all this, you need to follow simple and sustainable strength-training and nutrition programs that help you rack up consistent results over the long term.

As you strength train, try to create as much mechanical tension as possible while minimizing muscle damage and metabolic stress. By doing so, you will create the best stimuli for muscle growth.

Keep putting more and more stress on your body as it gets used to the stress you've already put on it. This will help you consistently build muscle and increase your strength as efficiently as possible.

Train your muscles through their full range of motion with constant tension and perfect technique, but don't train to the point of complete muscular failure.

Then, give your muscles enough time and fuel to recover by adjusting your training program based on your experience level, forming a routine that improves your biorhythm and recovery, and eating a quality diet.

Ensure that your diet is also satiating, prioritizes building muscle, and is adjusted based on your weight-change goals.

Fat gain and fat loss are primarily defined by calories in versus calories out. To lose excess body fat, you need to consume fewer calories than you burn, and to gain weight, you must consume more calories than you burn. Determine the number of calories you need to consume and burn based on your daily level of activity and your current body weight, and adjust your meal plan to work toward your weight-change goals.

To help with health and nutrient partitioning for optimal fat loss and muscle building, you need to eat the right foods in the right quantities. At a bare minimum, do your best to include fiber, high-quality protein sources, healthy dietary fats, and omega-3 fatty acids.

Add your favorite foods into your diet program to make it more sustainable, and get all your protein and other nutrients from whole foods before including other food sources.

You don't need protein shakes or other supplements unless you have trouble getting all the nutrients you need from your meals or you need a little extra help building muscle or losing fat.

When dieting, be sure to track your calories and macronutrients using a tracking target you can consistently hit so you can know that your diet is accurate and you will get results.

Also, make sure your body composition is changing the way that you want it to by routinely measuring your performance in the gym, how you are feeling mentally and physically, your body weight, and what you look like in photos.

Adjust your diet, training program, or routine based on your internal and external results.

Lastly, I hope you now understand that much of the information out there related to fat loss and muscle gain is based on the ideas of bro scientists and genetically blessed (or enhanced) fitness influencers, and most of the information is inaccurate.

If you focus on what we have gone over throughout *Physique Secrets*, you will be able to transform your body and keep getting results for life.

HELP ME HELP YOU BETTER

My goal is to cut through all the BS in the fitness and nutrition industries and provide every person with an affordable, high-quality education. There are too many people who get taken advantage of by awful trainers, coaches, companies, and marketers. If most people only had a basic understanding of what they needed to do, they could avoid the overwhelm and finally get results.

In order for me to continue to help you, I need to be able to keep writing books and improving the books that I've written thus far, based on what you need to know to succeed.

And in order for me to be able to keep educating you, I have to sell books. Without selling any books, unfortunately, I would not be able to make a living and have the free time to put life-changing information down onto pages.

So, if you enjoyed reading this book or learned something from it, please leave me a review and a rating on Amazon or on whatever platform or store you purchased this book from. This not only helps me keep lights on in my house and food on my table, but also helps me have time to help many people at once through education and more books. In addition, by leaving reviews and ratings, you can help someone else who might be struggling find this book and transform their life and body.

This industry runs on reviews, so your good word is immensely helpful, and I can't thank you enough if you do choose to take the time out of your day to drop a review and rating.

And if you didn't like the book, or you liked some parts and would want to see changes made in other parts, I would love to hear about that too! Honesty drives genuine improvement. I am constantly making updates to the book based on your feedback.

Finally, if you do leave a review, I can let you know when the next edition is available, when new books are released based on what you want to learn next, whether there are any discounts on books, or if changes have been made based on your recommendations.

If you have any questions about implementing the information or have ideas for other books you'd like to read in the future, please don't hesitate to reach out! You can do this by contacting me on social media.

Instagram: @iamnickschlager

Finally, I would love to see your transformation photos! Feel free to tag me in them or send them to me via social media or email.

Thank you, and good luck!

—Nick Schlager

REFERENCES

Chapter 2

1. Sørensen, T. I. A., Frederiksen, P. & Heitmann, B. L. (2020). Levels and changes in body mass index decomposed into fat and fat-free mass index: Relation to long-term all-cause mortality in the general population. International Journal of Obesity, 44, 2092–2100. https://doi.org/10.1038/s41366-020-0613-8

2. Kopelman, P. (2000). Obesity as a medical problem. Nature, 404, 635–643. https://doi.org/10.1038/35007508

3. Malmir, H., Mirzababaei, A., Moradi, S., Rezaei, S., Mirzaei, K. & Dadfarma, A. (2019). Metabolically healthy status and BMI in relation to depression: A systematic review of observational studies. Diabetes & Metabolic Syndrome: Clinical Research & Reviews, 13(2), 1099–1103. DOI: 10.1016/j.dsx.2019.01.027

4. Redman, L. M. & Ravussin, E. (2011). Caloric restriction in humans: Impact on physiological, psychological, and behavioral outcomes. Antioxidants & Redox Signaling, 14(2), 275–287. https://doi.org/10.1089/ars.2010.3253

5. Mattison, J. A., Colman, R. J., Beasley, T. M., Allison, D. B., Kemnitz, J. W., Roth, G. S., Ingram, D. K., Weindruch, R., de Cabo, R. & Anderson, R. M. (2017). Caloric restriction improves health and survival of rhesus monkeys. Nature Communications, 8, 14063. https://doi.org/10.1038/ncomms14063

6. Broskey, N. T., Marlatt, K. L., Most, J., Erickson, M. L., Irving, B. A. & Redman, L. M. (2019). The Panacea of Human Aging: Calorie Restriction Versus Exercise. Exercise and Sport Sciences Reviews, 47(3), 169–175. https://doi.org/10.1249/JES.0000000000000193

7. Cespedes Feliciano, E. M., Kroenke, C. H. & Caan, B. J. (2018). The Obesity Paradox in Cancer: How Important Is Muscle? Annual Review of Nutrition, 38, 357–379. https://doi.org/10.1146/annurev-nutr-082117-051723

8. Srikanthan, P. & Karlamangla, A. S. (2014). Muscle mass index as a predictor of longevity in older adults. American Journal of Medicine, 127(6), 547–553. https://doi.org/10.1016/j.amjmed.2014.02.007

9. Lampi, N. (2020, January 2). How to build an aesthetic Hollywood actor type physique: Complete guide. Iron Built Fitness. Retrieved from https://www.ironbuiltfitness.com/how-to-build-an-aesthetic-physique.

Chapter 3

1. Malmir, H., Mirzababaei, A., Moradi, S., Rezaei, S., Mirzaei, K. & Dadfarma, A. (2019). Metabolically healthy status and BMI in relation to depression: A systematic review of observational studies. Diabetes & Metabolic Syndrome: Clinical Research & Reviews, 13(2), 1099–1103. DOI: 10.1016/j.dsx.2019.01.027

2. Calle, M. C. & Fernandez, M. L. (2010). Effects of resistance training on the inflammatory response. Nutrition Research and Practice, 4(4), 259. DOI: 10.4162/nrp.2010.4.4.259

3. Saeidifard, F., Medina-Inojosa, J. R., West, C. P., Olson, T. P., Somers, V. K., Bonikowske, A. R., Prokop, L. J., Vinciguerra, M. & Lopez-Jimenez, F. (2019). The association of resistance training with mortality: A systematic review and meta-analysis. European Journal of Preventive Cardiology, 26(15), 1647–1665. DOI: 10.1177/2047487319850718

4. Brown, R. D. & Harrison, J. M. (1986). The effects of a strength training program on the strength and self-concept of two female age groups. Research Quarterly for Exercise and Sport, 57(4), 315–320. DOI: 10.1080/02701367.1986.10608092

5. Srikanthan, P. & Karlamangla, A. S. Relative Muscle Mass Is Inversely Associated with Insulin Resistance and Prediabetes. Findings from The Third National Health and Nutrition Examination Survey. Journal of Clinical Endocrinology & Metabolism, 96(9), 1 September 2011, 2898–2903. https://doi.org/10.1210/jc.2011-0435

6. Kopelman, P. (2000). Obesity as a medical problem. Nature, 404, 635–643. https://doi.org/10.1038/35007508

Chapter 4

1. Fryar, C. D., Carroll, M. D. & Afful, J. (2020). Prevalence of overweight, obesity, and severe obesity among adults aged 20 and over: United States, 1960–1962 through 2017–2018. NCHS Health E-Stats.

2. Booth, A. O., Wang, X., Turner, A. I., Nowson, C. A. & Torres, S. J. (2018). Diet-Induced Weight Loss Has No Effect on Psychological Stress in Overweight and Obese Adults: A Meta-Analysis of Randomized Controlled Trials. Nutrients, 10(5), 613. https://doi.org/10.3390/nu10050613

3. Attuquayefio, T. & Stevenson, R. J. (2015). A systematic review of longer-term dietary interventions on human cognitive function: Emerging patterns and future directions. Appetite, 95, 554–570. https://doi.org/10.1016/j.appet.2015.08.023

4. Mantantzis, K., Schlaghecken, F., Sünram-Lea, S. I. & Maylor, E. A. Sugar rush or sugar crash? A meta-analysis of carbohydrate effects on mood. Neuroscience & Biobehavioral Reviews, 101, 2019, 45–67. ISSN 0149-7634. https://doi.org/10.1016/j.neubiorev.2019.03.016

5. Solianik, R., Sujeta, A., Terentjevienė, A. & Skurvydas, A. (2016). Effect of 48 h Fasting on Autonomic Function, Brain Activity, Cognition, and Mood in Amateur Weight Lifters. BioMed Research International, 2016, 1503956. https://doi.org/10.1155/2016/1503956

Chapter 5

1. West, D. W., Burd, N. A., Staples, A. W. & Phillips, S. M. (2010). Human exercise-mediated skeletal muscle hypertrophy is an intrinsic process. International Journal of Biochemistry & Cell Biology, 42(9), 1371–1375. DOI: 10.1016/j.biocel.2010.05.012

2. Colliander, E. B. & Tesch, P. A. (1990). Effects of eccentric and concentric muscle actions in resistance training. Acta Physiologica Scandinavica, 140(1), 31–39. DOI: 10.1111/j.1748-1716.1990.tb08973.x

3. Heather, B. M., Tesch, P. A., Buchanan, P. & Dudley, G. A. (1991). Influence of eccentric actions on skeletal muscle adaptations to resistance training. Acta Physiologica Scandinavica, 143(2), 177–185. DOI: 10.1111/j.1748-1716.1991.tb09219.x

4. Tesch, P. A., Thorsson, A. & Colliander, E. B. (1990). Effects of eccentric and concentric resistance training on skeletal muscle substrates, enzyme activities and capillary supply. Acta Physiologica Scandinavica, 140(4), 575–579. DOI: 10.1111/j.1748-1716.1990.tb09035.x

5. Bjørnsen, T., Wernbom, M., Løvstad, A., Paulsen, G., D'Souza, R. F., Cameron-Smith, D., Flesche, A., Hisdal, J., Berntsen, S. & Raastad, T. (2019). Delayed myonuclear addition, myofiber hypertrophy, and increases in strength with high-frequency low-load blood flow restricted training to volitional failure. Journal of Applied Physiology, 126(3), 578–592. DOI: 10.1152/japplphysiol.00397.2018

6. Longo, A. R., Silva-Batista, C., Pedroso, K., de Salles Painelli, V., Lasevicius, T., Schoenfeld, B. J., Aihara, A. Y., de Almeida Peres, B., Tricoli, V. & Teixeira, E. L. Volume Load Rather Than Resting Interval Influences Muscle Hypertrophy During High-Intensity Resistance Training. Journal of Strength and Conditioning Research, 36(6), June 2022. 1554–1559. DOI: 10.1519/JSC.0000000000003668

7. Schoenfeld, B. J., Ratamess, N. A., Peterson, M. D., Contreras, B., Sonmez, G. T. & Alvar, B. A. (2014). Effects of different volume-equated resistance training loading strategies on muscular adaptations in well-trained men. Journal of Strength and Conditioning Research, 28(10), 2909–2918. https://doi.org/10.1519/JSC.0000000000000480

8. Heymsfield, S. B., Stevens, V., Noel, R., McManus, C., Smith, J. & Nixon, D. Biochemical composition of muscle in normal and semistarved human subjects: relevance to anthropometric measurements. American Journal of Clinical Nutrition, 36(1), July 1982, 131–142. https://doi.org/10.1093/ajcn/36.1.131

9. Vehrs, P. & Hager, R. (2006). Assessment and Interpretation of Body Composition in Physical Education, Journal of Physical Education, Recreation & Dance, 77(7), 46–51. DOI: 10.1080/07303084.2006.10597907

10. Pallarés, J. G., Martínez-Abellán, A., López-Gullón, J. M., Morán-Navarro, R., De la Cruz-Sánchez, E. & Mora-Rodríguez, R. (2016). Muscle contraction velocity, strength and power output changes following different degrees of hypohydration in competitive Olympic combat sports. Journal of the International Society of Sports Nutrition, 13, 10. https://doi.org/10.1186/s12970-016-0121-3

11. Dattilo, M., Antunes, H., Medeiros, A., Mônico Neto, M., Souza, H., Tufik, S. & de Mello, M. (2011). Sleep and muscle recovery: Endocrinological and molecular basis for a new and promising hypothesis. Medical Hypotheses, 77(2), 220–222. DOI: 10.1016/j.mehy.2011.04.017

12. Amstrup, A. K., Sikjaer, T., Pedersen, S. B., Heickendorff, L., Mosekilde, L. & Rejnmark, L. (2016). Reduced fat mass and increased lean mass in response to 1 year of melatonin treatment in postmenopausal women: A randomized placebo-controlled trial. Clinical Endocrinology, 84(3), 342–347. https://doi.org/10.1111/cen.12942

13. Prather, A. A., Epel, E. S., Arenander, J., Broestl, L., Garay, B. I., Wang, D. & Dubal, D. B. (2015). Longevity factor klotho and chronic psychological stress. Translational Psychiatry, 5(6), e585. https://doi.org/10.1038/tp.2015.81

14. Stults-Kolehmainen, M. A., Bartholomew, J. B. & Sinha, R. (2014). Chronic psychological stress impairs recovery of muscular function and somatic sensations over a 96-hour period. Journal of Strength and Conditioning Research, 28(7), 2007–2017. https://doi.org/10.1519/JSC.0000000000000335

15. Quintero, K. J., Resende, A., Leite, G. S. F., et al. (2018). An overview of nutritional strategies for recovery process in sports-related muscle injuries. Nutrire, 43, 27. https://doi.org/10.1186/s41110-018-0084-z

Chapter 6

1. Demling, R. H. & DeSanti, L. (2000). Effect of a hypocaloric diet, increased protein intake and resistance training on lean mass gains and fat mass loss in overweight police officers. Annals of Nutrition and Metabolism, 44(1), 21–29. DOI: 10.1159/000012817

2. Josse, A. R., Tang, J. E., Tarnopolsky, M. A. & Phillips, S. M. (2010). Body composition and strength changes in women with milk and resistance exercise. Medicine & Science in Sports & Exercise, 42(6), 1122–1130. DOI: 10.1249/mss.0b013e3181c854f6

3. Nindl, B. C., Harman, E. A., Marx, J. O., Gotshalk, L. A., Frykman, P. N., Lammi, E., Palmer, C. & Kraemer, W. J. (2000). Regional body composition changes in women after 6 months of periodized physical training. Journal of Applied Physiology, 88(6), 2251–2259. DOI: 10.1152/jappl.2000.88.6.2251

4. Garthe, I., Raastad, T., Refsnes, P. E., Koivisto, A. & Sundgot-Borgen, J. (2011). Effect of two different weight-loss rates on body composition and strength and power-related performance in elite athletes. International Journal of Sport Nutrition and Exercise Metabolism, 21(2), 97–104. DOI: 10.1123/ijsnem.21.2.97

5. Davidsen, P. K., Gallagher, I. J., Hartman, J. W., Tarnopolsky, M. A., Dela, F., Helge, J. W., Timmons, J. A. & Phillips, S. M. (2011). High responders to resistance exercise training demonstrate differential regulation of skeletal muscle microRNA expression. Journal of Applied Physiology, 110(2), 309–317. DOI: 10.1152/japplphysiol.00901.2010

6. Ariel, G. & Saville, W. (1972). Anabolic steroids: The physiological effects of placebos. Medicine & Science in Sports & Exercise, 4, 124–6.

7. Zempo, H., Miyamoto-Mikami, E., Kikuchi, N., Fuku, N., Miyachi, M. & Murakami, H. (2016). Heritability estimates of muscle strength-related phenotypes: A systematic review and meta-analysis. Scandinavian Journal of Medicine & Science in Sports, 27(12), 1537–1546. DOI: 10.1111/sms.12804

8. Mobley, C. B., Haun, C. T., Roberson, P. A., Mumford, P. W., Kephart, W. C., et al. (2018). Biomarkers associated with low, moderate, and high vastus lateralis muscle hypertrophy following 12 weeks of resistance training. PLOS ONE 13(4), e0195203. https://doi.org/10.1371/journal.pone.0195203

9. Walker, S., Taipale, R. S., Nyman, K., Kraemer, W. J. & Häkkinen, K. (2011). Neuromuscular and hormonal responses to constant and variable resistance loadings. Medicine & Science in Sports & Exercise, 43(1), 26–33. DOI: 10.1249/mss.0b013e3181e71bcb

10. Keogh, J. W. & Winwood, P. W. (2017). The Epidemiology of Injuries across the Weight-Training Sports. Sports Medicine (Auckland, N.Z.), 47(3), 479–501. https://doi.org/10.1007/s40279-016-0575-0

11. McCaw, S. T. & Friday, J. J. (1994). A comparison of muscle activity between a free weight and machine bench press. Journal of Strength and Conditioning Research, 8(4), 259–264. DOI: 10.1519/00124278-199411000-00011

12. Schwanbeck, S. R., Cornish, S. M., Barss, T. & Chilibeck, P. D. (2020). Effects of training with free weights versus machines on muscle mass, strength, free testosterone, and free cortisol levels. Journal of Strength and Conditioning Research, 34(7), 1851–1859. DOI: 10.1519/jsc.0000000000003349

13. Schott, N., Johnen, B. & Holfelder, B. (2019). Effects of free weights and machine training on muscular strength in high-functioning older adults. Experimental Gerontology, 122, 15–24. DOI: 10.1016/j.exger.2019.03.012

14. Heron, M. I. & Richmond, F. J. (1993). In-series fiber architecture in long human muscles. Journal of Morphology, 216(1), 35–45. https://doi.org/10.1002/jmor.1052160106

15. Mendiguchia, J., Garrues, M. A., Cronin, J. B., Contreras, B., Los Arcos, A., Malliaropoulos, N., Maffulli, N. & Idoate, F. (2013). Nonuniform changes in MRI measurements of the thigh muscles after two hamstring strengthening exercises. Journal of Strength and Conditioning Research, 27(3), 574–581. https://doi.org/10.1519/JSC.0b013e31825c2f38

16. Kubota, J., Ono, T., Araki, M., Torii, S., Okuwaki, T. & Fukubayashi, T. (2007). Non-uniform changes in magnetic resonance measurements of the semitendinosus muscle following intensive eccentric exercise. European Journal of Applied Physiology, 101(6), 713–720. https://doi.org/10.1007/s00421-007-0549-x

17. Stokes, T., Hector, A. J., Morton, R. W., McGlory, C. & Phillips, S. M. (2018). Recent Perspectives Regarding the Role of Dietary Protein for the Promotion of Muscle Hypertrophy with Resistance Exercise Training. Nutrients, 10(2),180. https://doi.org/10.3390/nu10020180

18. Morton, R. W., Murphy, K. T., McKellar, S. R., Schoenfeld, B. J., Henselmans, M., Helms, E., Aragon, A. A., Devries, M. C., Banfield, L., Krieger, J. W. & Phillips, S. M. (2017). A systematic review, meta-analysis and meta-regression of the effect of protein supplementation on resistance

training-induced gains in muscle mass and strength in healthy adults. British Journal of Sports Medicine, 52(6), 376–384. DOI: 10.1136/bjsports-2017-097608

19. Roberts, J., Zinchenko, A., Suckling, C., Smith, L., Johnstone, J. & Henselmans, M. (2017). The short-term effect of high versus moderate protein intake on recovery after strength training in resistance-trained individuals. Journal of the International Society of Sports Nutrition, 14(1). DOI: 10.1186/s12970-017-0201-z

20. Tarnopolsky, M. A., Atkinson, S. A., MacDougall, J. D., Chesley, A., Phillips, S. & Schwarcz, H. P. (1992). Evaluation of protein requirements for trained strength athletes. Journal of Applied Physiology, 73(5), 1986–1995. DOI: 10.1152/jappl.1992.73.5.1986

21. Da Silva, R. L., Brentano, M. A. & Kruel, L. F. (2010). Effects of different strength training methods on postexercise energetic expenditure. Journal of Strength and Conditioning Research, 24(8), 2255–60. DOI: 10.1519/JSC.0b013e3181aff2ba

22. Brentano, M. A., Umpierre, D., Santos, L. P., Lopes, A. L. & Kruel, L. F. M. (2016). Supersets do not change energy expenditure during strength training sessions in physically active individuals. Journal of Exercise Science & Fitness, 14(2), 41–46. DOI: 10.1016/j.jesf.2016.05.003.

23. Alcaraz, P. E., Perez-Gomez, J., Chavarrias, M. & Blazevich, A. J. Similarity in adaptations to high-resistance circuit vs. traditional strength training in resistance-trained men. Journal of Strength and Conditioning Research, 25(9), 2519–27. DOI: 10.1519/JSC.0b013e3182023a51

Chapter 7

1. Zeng, Q., Dong, S. Y., Sun, X. N., Xie, J. & Cui, Y. (2012). Percent body fat is a better predictor of cardiovascular risk factors than body mass index. Brazilian Journal of Medical and Biological Research, 45(7), 591–600. DOI: 10.1590/s0100-879x2012007500059

2. Hruby, A. & Hu, F. B. (2014). The epidemiology of obesity: A big picture. PharmacoEconomics, 33(7), 673–689. DOI: 10.1007/s40273-014-0243-x

3. Halton, T. L. & Hu, F. B. (2004). The Effects of High Protein Diets on Thermogenesis, Satiety and Weight Loss: A Critical Review. Journal of the American College of Nutrition, 23(5), 373–385. DOI: 10.1080/07315724.2004.10719381

4. Cunningham, J. J. (1991). Body composition as a determinant of energy expenditure: A synthetic review and a proposed general prediction equation. American Journal of Clinical Nutrition, 54(6), 963–969. DOI: 10.1093/ajcn/54.6.963

5. Reynolds, A., Mann, J., Cummings, J., Winter, N., Mete, E. & te Morenga, L. (2019). Carbohydrate quality and human health: A series of systematic reviews and meta-analyses. Lancet, 393(10170), 434–445. DOI: 10.1016/s0140-6736(18)31809-9

6. Slavin, J. L. & Lloyd, B. (2012). Health benefits of fruits and vegetables. Advances in Nutrition (Bethesda, Md.), 3(4), 506–516. https://doi.org/10.3945/an.112.002154

7. Blanchflower, D., Oswald, A. & Stewart-Brown, S. (2013). Is Psychological Well-Being Linked to the Consumption of Fruit and Vegetables? Social Indicators Research: An International and

Interdisciplinary Journal for Quality-of-Life Measurement, Springer, 114(3), 785–801. DOI: 10.3386/w18469

8. Riechman, S. E., Andrews, R. D., MacLean, D. A. & Sheather, S. Authors' Response to Lambert Letter on Saturated Fat Ingestion. Journals of Gerontology: Series A, 63(11), November 2008, 1260–1261. https://doi.org/10.1093/gerona/63.11.1260-a

9. Gromadzka-Ostrowska, J. (2006). Effects of dietary fat on androgen secretion and metabolism. Reproductive Biology, 6 Suppl 2, 13–20. PMID: 17220937

10. Ingram, D. M., Bennett, F. C., Willcox, D. & de Klerk, N. (1987). Effect of low-fat diet on female sex hormone levels. Journal of the National Cancer Institute, 79(6), 1225–1229.

11. Volek, J. S., Kraemer, W. J., Bush, J. A., Incledon, T. & Boetes, M. (1997). Testosterone and cortisol in relationship to dietary nutrients and resistance exercise. Journal of Applied Physiology, 82(1), 49–54. DOI: 10.1152/jappl.1997.82.1.49

12. Dorgan, J. F., Judd, J. T., Longcope, C., Brown, C., Schatzkin, A., Clevidence, B. A., Campbell, W. S., Nair, P. P., Franz, C., Kahle, L. & Taylor, P. R. Effects of dietary fat and fiber on plasma and urine androgens and estrogens in men: A controlled feeding study. American Journal of Clinical Nutrition, 64(6), December 1996, 850–855. https://doi.org/10.1093/ajcn/64.6.850

13. Wittert, G. A., Chapman, I. M., Haren, M. T., Mackintosh, S., Coates, P. & Morley, J. E. Oral testosterone supplementation increases muscle and decreases fat mass in healthy elderly males with low-normal gonadal status. Journals of Gerontology Series A, Biological Sciences and Medical Sciences, 58(7), July 2003, 618–25. DOI: 10.1093/gerona/58.7.m618. PMID: 12865477

14. Yeo, J. K., Cho, S. I., Park, S. G., Jo, S., Ha, J. K., Lee, J. W., Cho, S. Y. & Park, M. G. Which Exercise Is Better for Increasing Serum Testosterone Levels in Patients with Erectile Dysfunction? World Journal of Men's Health, 36(2), May 2018, 147–152. DOI: 10.5534/wjmh.17030. Epub 2018 Jan 26. PMID: 29623694; PMCID: PMC5924956

15. Rosqvist, F., Iggman, D., Kullberg, J., Cedernaes, J., Johansson, H. E., Larsson, A., Johansson, L., Ahlström, H., Arner, P., Dahlman, I. & Risérus, U. Overfeeding polyunsaturated and saturated fat causes distinct effects on liver and visceral fat accumulation in humans. Diabetes, 63(7), July 2014, 2356–2368. DOI: 10.2337/db13-1622. Epub 2014 Feb 18. PMID: 24550191

16. Accardi, G., Aiello, A., Gargano, V., et al. (2016). Nutraceutical effects of table green olives: A pilot study with Nocellara del Belice olives. Immunity & Ageing 13, 11. https://doi.org/10.1186/s12979-016-0067-y

17. Smith, G. I., Atherton, P., Reeds, D. N., Mohammed, B. S., Rankin, D., Rennie, M. J. & Mittendorfer, B. Omega-3 polyunsaturated fatty acids augment the muscle protein anabolic response to hyperinsulinaemia-hyperaminoacidaemia in healthy young and middle-aged men and women. Clinical Science (London), 121(6), September 2011, 267–278. DOI: 10.1042/CS20100597. PMID: 21501117; PMCID: PMC3499967

18. Logan, S. L. & Spriet, L. L. (2015, December 17). Omega-3 fatty acid supplementation for 12 weeks increases resting and exercise metabolic rate in healthy community-dwelling older females. PLOS ONE, 10(12). DOI: 10.1371/journal.pone.0144828

19. Couet, C., Delarue, J., Ritz, P., Antoine, J. M. & Lamisse, F. Effect of dietary fish oil on body fat mass and basal fat oxidation in healthy adults. International Journal of Obesity and Related Metabolic Disorders, 21(8), August 1997, 637–643. DOI: 10.1038/sj.ijo.0800451

20. Corder, K., Newsham, K., McDaniel, J., Caciano, S., Ezekiel, U., Sisler, C. & Weiss, E. (2014). Effects of short-term docosahexaenoic acid supplementation on markers of inflammation after eccentric strength exercise. Journal of the Academy of Nutrition and Dietetics, 114(9), A63. DOI: 10.1016/j.jand.2014.06.209

21. Wani, A. L., Bhat, S. A. & Ara, A. (2015). Omega-3 fatty acids and the treatment of depression: a review of scientific evidence. Integrative Medicine Research, 4(3), 132–141. DOI: 10.1016/j.imr.2015.07.003

22. Huang, Y. H., Chiu, W. C., Hsu, Y. P., Lo, Y. L. & Wang, Y. H. (2020). Effects of omega-3 fatty acids on muscle mass, muscle strength and muscle performance among the elderly: A meta-analysis. Nutrients, 12(12), 3739. DOI: 10.3390/nu12123739

23. Volek, J. S., Kraemer, W. J., Bush, J. A., Incledon, T., & Boetes, M. (1997). Testosterone and cortisol in relationship to dietary nutrients and resistance exercise. Journal of Applied Physiology, 82(1), 49–54. DOI: 10.1152/jappl.1997.82.1.49

24. Gerling, C. J., Whitfield, J., Mukai, K. & Spriet, L. L. (2014). Variable effects of 12 weeks of omega-3 supplementation on resting skeletal muscle metabolism. Applied Physiology, Nutrition, and Metabolism, 39(9), 1083–1091. DOI: 10.1139/apnm-2014-0049

25. Lepretti, M., Martucciello, S., Burgos Aceves, M., Putti, R. & Lionetti, L. (2018). Omega-3 fatty acids and insulin resistance: Focus on the regulation of mitochondria and endoplasmic reticulum stress. Nutrients, 10(3), 350. DOI: 10.3390/nu10030350

26. Johnson, G. H. & Fritsche, K. (2012). Effect of Dietary Linoleic Acid on Markers of Inflammation in Healthy Persons: A Systematic Review of Randomized Controlled Trials. Journal of the Academy of Nutrition and Dietetics, 112(7), 1029–1041.e15. https://doi.org/10.1016/j.jand.2012.03.029

Chapter 8

1. Forbes, G. B. (2006). Body fat content influences the body composition response to nutrition and exercise. Annals of the New York Academy of Sciences, 904(1), 359–365. DOI: 10.1111/j.1749-6632.2000.tb06482.x

2. Swaminathan, R., King, R. F., Holmfield, J., Siwek, R. A., Baker, M. & Wales, J. K. (1985). Thermic effect of feeding carbohydrate, fat, protein and mixed meal in lean and obese subjects. American Journal of Clinical Nutrition, 42(2), 177–181. DOI: 10.1093/ajcn/42.2.177

3. Müller, M. J., Geisler, C., Heymsfield, S. B. & Bosy-Westphal, A. (2018). Recent advances in understanding body weight homeostasis in humans. F1000Research, 7, 1025. DOI: 10.12688/f1000research.14151.1

4. Hartmann-Boyce, J., Johns, D. J., Jebb, S. A. & Aveyard, P. (2014). Effect of behavioural techniques and delivery mode on effectiveness of weight management: systematic review, meta-analysis and meta-regression. Obesity Reviews, 15(7), 598–609. DOI: 10.1111/obr.12165

5. Peterson, N. D., Middleton, K. R., Nackers, L. M., Medina, K. E., Milsom, V. A. & Perri, M. G. (2014). Dietary self-monitoring and long-term success with weight management. Obesity, 22(9), 1962–1967. https://doi.org/10.1002/oby.20807

6. Goldstein, S. P., Goldstein, C. M., Bond, D. S., Raynor, H. A., Wing, R. R. & Thomas, J. G. (2019). Associations between self-monitoring and weight change in behavioral weight loss interventions. Health Psychology, 38(12), 1128–1136. DOI: 10.1037/hea0000800

7. Patel, M. L., Wakayama, L. N. & Bennett, G. G. (2021). Self-monitoring via digital health in weight loss interventions: A systematic review among adults with overweight or obesity. Obesity, 29(3), 478–499. DOI: 10.1002/oby.23088

8. Kelley, C. P., Sbrocco, G. & Sbrocco, T. (2016). Behavioral modification for the management of obesity. Primary Care: Clinics in Office Practice, 43(1), 159–175. DOI: 10.1016/j.pop.2015.10.004

9. Wajchenberg, B. L. (2000). Subcutaneous and visceral adipose tissue: Their relation to the metabolic syndrome. Endocrine Reviews, 21(6), 697–738. https://doi.org/10.1210/edrv.21.6.0415

10. Bouchard, C., Tchernof, A. & Tremblay, A. (2014). Predictors of body composition and body energy changes in response to chronic overfeeding. International Journal of Obesity, 38, 236–242. https://doi.org/10.1038/ijo.2013.77

11. Saris, W., Astrup, A., Prentice, A., Zunft, H., Formiguera, X., Verboeket-van De Venne, W., Raben, A., Poppitt, S., Seppelt, B., Johnston, S., Vasilaras, T. & Keogh, G. (2000). Randomized controlled trial of changes in dietary carbohydrate/fat ratio and simple vs complex carbohydrates on body weight and blood lipids: The CARMEN study. International Journal of Obesity, 24(10), 1310–1318. DOI: /10.1038/sj.ijo.0801451

12. Gatenby, S. J., Aaron, J. I., Jack, V. A. & Mela, D. J. (1997). Extended use of foods modified in fat and sugar content: Nutritional implications in a free-living female population. American Journal of Clinical Nutrition, 65(6), 1867–1873. DOI: 10.1093/ajcn/65.6.1867

13. Surwit, R. S., Feinglos, M. N., McCaskill, C. C., Clay, S. L., Babyak, M. A., Brownlow, B. S., Plaisted, C. S. & Lin, P. H. (1997). Metabolic and behavioral effects of a high-sucrose diet during weight loss. American Journal of Clinical Nutrition, 65(4), 908–915. DOI: 10.1093/ajcn/65.4.908

14. Vermunt, S. H. F., Pasman, W. J., Schaafsma, G. & Kardinaal, A. F. M. (2003). Effects of sugar intake on body weight: a review. Obesity Reviews, 4(2), 91–99. DOI: 10.1046/j.1467-789x.2003.00102.x

15. West, J. & de Looy, A. (2001). Weight loss in overweight subjects following low-sucrose or sucrose-containing diets. International Journal of Obesity, 25(8), 1122–1128. DOI: 10.1038/sj.ijo.0801652

16. Hu, T., Mills, K. T., Yao, L., Demanelis, K., Eloustaz, M., Yancy, W. S., Kelly, T. N., He, J. & Bazzano, L. A. (2012). Effects of low-carbohydrate diets versus low-fat diets on metabolic risk factors: A meta-analysis of randomized controlled clinical trials. American Journal of Epidemiology, 176(7), S44–S54. DOI: 10.1093/aje/kws264

17. Tobias, D. K., Chen, M., Manson, J. E., Ludwig, D. S., Willett, W. & Hu, F. B. (2015). Effect of low-fat diet interventions versus other diet interventions on long-term weight change in adults: A systematic review and meta-analysis. Lancet Diabetes & Endocrinology, 3(12), 968–979. DOI: 10.1016/s2213-8587(15)00367-8

18. Nordmann, A. J., Nordmann, A., Briel, M., Keller, U., Yancy, W. S., Brehm, B. J. & Bucher, H. C. (2006). Effects of Low-Carbohydrate vs Low-Fat Diets on Weight Loss and Cardiovascular Risk Factors. Archives of Internal Medicine, 166(3), 285. https://doi.org/10.1001/archinte.166.3.285

19. Hirsch, J., Hudgins, L. C., Leibel, R. L. & Rosenbaum, M. (1998). Diet composition and energy balance in humans. American Journal of Clinical Nutrition, 67(3), 551S–555S. DOI: 10.1093/ajcn/67.3.551s

20. Crestani, D. M., Bonin, É. F. R., Barbieri, R. A., et al. (2017). Chronic supplementation of omega-3 can improve body composition and maximal strength, but does not change the resistance to neuromuscular fatigue. Sport Sciences for Health, 13, 259–265. https://doi.org/10.1007/s11332-016-0322-9

21. Logan, S. L. & Spriet, L. L. (2015, December 17). Omega-3 fatty acid supplementation for 12 weeks increases resting and exercise metabolic rate in healthy community-dwelling older females. PLOS ONE, 10(12). DOI: 10.1371/journal.pone.0144828

22. Fox, D. M., Martin, A. R., Murphy, C. A. & Koehler, K. (2019). Contribution of changes in body composition and adaptive thermogenesis to the decline in resting metabolic rate during prolonged calorie-restricted weight loss. FASEB Journal, 33, 699.2–699.2. DOI: 10.1096/fasebj.2019.33.1_supplement.699.2

23. Hintze, L. J., Goldfield, G., Seguin, R., Damphousse, A., Riopel, A. & Doucet, É. (2019). The rate of weight loss does not affect resting energy expenditure and appetite sensations differently in women living with overweight and obesity. Physiology & Behavior, 199, 314–321. DOI: 10.1016/j.physbeh.2018.11.032

24. Ostendorf, D. M., Melanson, E. L., Caldwell, A. E., Creasy, S. A., Pan, Z., MacLean, P. S., Wyatt, H. R., Hill, J. O. & Catenacci, V. A. (2018). No consistent evidence of a disproportionately low resting energy expenditure in long-term successful weight-loss maintainers. American Journal of Clinical Nutrition, 108(4), 658–666. DOI: 10.1093/ajcn/nqy179

25. Zinchenko, A. & Henselmans, M. (2016). Metabolic damage: Do negative metabolic adaptations during underfeeding persist after refeeding in non-obese populations? Medical Research Archives, 4(8). ISSN: 2375-1924

26. Clark, J. E. (2015). Diet, exercise or diet with exercise: Comparing the effectiveness of treatment options for weight-loss and changes in fitness for adults (18-65 years old) who are overfat, or obese; systematic review and meta-analysis. Journal of Diabetes and Metabolic Disorders, 14, 31. https://doi.org/10.1186/s40200-015-0154-1

27. Skelly, L. E., Andrews, P. C., Gillen, J. B., Martin, B. J., Percival, M. E. & Gibala, M. J. (2014). High-intensity interval exercise induces 24-h energy expenditure similar to traditional endurance exercise despite reduced time commitment. Applied Physiology, Nutrition, and Metabolism, 39(7), 845–848. DOI: 10.1139/apnm-2013-0562

28. Cunningham, J. J. (1991). Body composition as a determinant of energy expenditure: A synthetic review and a proposed general prediction equation. American Journal of Clinical Nutrition, 54(6), 963–969. DOI: 10.1093/ajcn/54.6.963

29. Strasser, B., Spreitzer, A. & Haber, P. (2007). Fat loss depends on energy deficit only, independently of the method for weight loss. Annals of Nutrition & Metabolism, 51(5), 428–432. https://doi.org/10.1159/000111162

30. Donnelly, J. E., Herrmann, S. D., Lambourne, K., Szabo, A. N., Honas, J. J. & Washburn, R. A. (2014). Does increased exercise or physical activity alter ad-libitum daily energy intake or macronutrient composition in healthy adults? A systematic review. PloS One, 9(1), e83498. https://doi.org/10.1371/journal.pone.0083498

31. Shakiba, E., Sheikholeslami-Vatani, D., Rostamzadeh, N. & Karim, H. The type of training program affects appetite-regulating hormones and body weight in overweight sedentary men. Applied Physiology, Nutrition, and Metabolism, 44(3): 282–287. https://doi.org/10.1139/apnm-2018-0197

32. Thivel, D., Aucouturier, J., Metz, L., Morio, B. & Duché, P. (2014). Is there spontaneous energy expenditure compensation in response to intensive exercise in obese youth? Pediatric Obesity, 9(2), 147–154. https://doi.org/10.1111/j.2047-6310.2013.00148.x

33. Shakiba, E., Sheikholeslami-Vatani, D., Rostamzadeh, N. & Karim, H. The type of training program affects appetite-regulating hormones and body weight in overweight sedentary men. Applied Physiology, Nutrition, and Metabolism, 44(3): 282–287. https://doi.org/10.1139/apnm-2018-0197

34. Thorogood, A., Mottillo, S., Shimony, A., Filion, K. B., Joseph, L., Genest, J., Pilote, L., Poirier, P., Schiffrin, E. L. & Eisenberg, M. J. (2011). Isolated Aerobic Exercise and Weight Loss: A Systematic Review and Meta-Analysis of Randomized Controlled Trials. American Journal of Medicine, 124(8), 747–755. ISSN 0002-9343. https://doi.org/10.1016/j.amjmed.2011.02.037

35. Dallosso, H. M., Murgatroyd, P. R. & James, W. P. (1982). Feeding frequency and energy balance in adult males. Human Nutrition: Clinical Nutrition, 36C(1), 25–39. PMID: 7076516

Chapter 10

1. Haaf, T. & Weijs, P. J. M. (2014). Resting energy expenditure prediction in recreational athletes of 18–35 years: Confirmation of Cunningham equation and an improved weight-based alternative. PLOS ONE 9(10). DOI: 10.1371/journal.pone.0108460

Chapter 11

1. Morton, R. W., Murphy, K. T., McKellar, S. R., Schoenfeld, B. J., Henselmans, M., Helms, E., Aragon, A. A., Devries, M. C., Banfield, L., Krieger, J. W. & Phillips, S. M. (2017). A systematic review, meta-analysis and meta-regression of the effect of protein supplementation on resistance training-induced gains in muscle mass and strength in healthy adults. British Journal of Sports Medicine, 52(6), 376–384. DOI: 10.1136/bjsports-2017-097608

2. Phillips, S. M. & van Loon, L. J. (2011). Dietary protein for athletes: From requirements to optimum adaptation. Journal of Sports Sciences, 29 (sup1), S29–S38. DOI: 10.1080/02640414.2011.619204

3. Carlton, A. & Orr, R. M. (2015). The effects of fluid loss on physical performance: A critical review. Journal of Sport and Health Science, 4(4), 357–363. ISSN 2095-2546. https://doi.org/10.1016/j.jshs.2014.09.004

4. McKinley, J. & Johnson, A. K. (2004). The Physiological Regulation of Thirst and Fluid Intake. American Physiological Society, 19(1), 1–6. DOI: 10.1152/nips.01470.2003

5. Hoffman, M. D., Bross III, T. L. & Hamilton, R. T. (2016). Are we being drowned by over-rhydration advice on the Internet? Physician and Sportsmedicine, 44(4), 343–348. DOI: 10.1080/00913847.2016.1222853

6. Kenefick, R. W. (2018). Drinking Strategies: Planned Drinking versus Drinking to Thirst. Sports Medicine, 48, 31–37. https://doi.org/10.1007/s40279-017-0844-6

7. Judelson, D. A., Maresh, C. M., Anderson, J. M., Armstrong, L. E., Casa, D. J., Kraemer, W. J. & Volek, J. S. (2007). Hydration and muscular performance: Does fluid balance affect strength, power and high-intensity endurance? Sports Medicine (Auckland, N.Z.), 37(10), 907–921. https://doi.org/10.2165/00007256-200737100-00006

Chapter 12

1. Anderson, J. W., Baird, P., Davis Jr., R. H., Ferreri, S., Knudtson, M., Koraym, A., Waters, V. & Williams, C. L. (2009). Health benefits of dietary fiber. Nutrition Reviews, 67(4), 188–205. DOI: 10.1111/j.1753-4887.2009.00189.x

2. Reynolds, A., Mann, J., Cummings, J., Winter, N., Mete, E. & te Morenga, L. (2019). Carbohydrate quality and human health: A series of systematic reviews and meta-analyses. Lancet, 393(10170), 434–445. DOI: 10.1016/s0140-6736(18)31809-9

3. Simopoulos, A. (2002). The importance of the ratio of omega-6/omega-3 essential fatty acids. Biomedicine & Pharmacotherapy, 56(8), 365–379. DOI: 10.1016/s0753-3322(02)00253-6

4. Johnson, G. H. & Fritsche, K. (2012). Effect of Dietary Linoleic Acid on Markers of Inflammation in Healthy Persons: A Systematic Review of Randomized Controlled Trials. Journal of the Academy of Nutrition and Dietetics, 112(7), 1029–1041.e15. https://doi.org/10.1016/j.jand.2012.03.029

5. Smith, G. I., Atherton, P., Reeds, D. N., Mohammed, B. S., Rankin, D., Rennie, M. J. & Mittendorfer, B. Omega-3 polyunsaturated fatty acids augment the muscle protein anabolic response to hyperinsulinaemia-hyperaminoacidaemia in healthy young and middle-aged men and women. Clinical Science (London), 121(6), September 2011, 267–278. doi: 10.1042/CS20100597. PMID: 21501117; PMCID: PMC3499967

6. Jeromson, S., Gallagher, I., Galloway, S. & Hamilton, D. (2015). Omega-3 Fatty Acids and Skeletal Muscle Health. Marine Drugs, 13(11), 6977–7004. https://doi.org/10.3390/md13116977

7. de Souza, R. J., Mente, A., Maroleanu, A., Cozma, A. I., Ha, V., Kishibe, T., Uleryk, E., Budylowski, P., Schünemann, H., Beyene, J. & Anand, S. S. (2015). Intake of saturated and trans unsaturated fatty acids and risk of all cause mortality, cardiovascular disease, and type 2 diabetes: Systematic review and meta-analysis of observational studies. BMJ, h3978. DOI: 10.1136/bmj.h3978

8. Hamley, S. (2017). The effect of replacing saturated fat with mostly n-6 polyunsaturated fat on coronary heart disease: A meta-analysis of randomised controlled trials. Nutrition Journal, 16(1). DOI: 10.1186/s12937-017-0254-5

9. Weinberg, S. L. (2004). The diet-heart hypothesis: A critique. Journal of the American College of Cardiology, 43(5), 731–733. DOI: 10.1016/j.jacc.2003.10.034

10. Morris, J. N., Marr, J. W., Heady, J. A., Mills, G. L. & Pilkington, T. R. E. (1963). Diet and plasma cholesterol in 99 bank men. BMJ, 1(5330), 571–576. DOI: 10.1136/bmj.1.5330.571

11. Shih, C. W., Hauser, M. E., Aronica, L., Rigdon, J. & Gardner, C. D. (2019). Changes in blood lipid concentrations associated with changes in intake of dietary saturated fat in the context of a healthy low-carbohydrate weight-loss diet: A secondary analysis of the Diet Intervention Examining The Factors Interacting with Treatment Success (DIETFITS) trial. American Journal of Clinical Nutrition, 109(2), 433–441. DOI: 10.1093/ajcn/nqy305

12. Blesso, C. N. & Fernandez, M. L. (2018). Dietary Cholesterol, Serum Lipids, and Heart Disease: Are Eggs Working for or against You? Nutrients, 10(4), 426. https://doi.org/10.3390/nu10040426

Chapter 13

1. Krings, B. M., Rountree, J. A., McAllister, M. J., et al. (2016). Effects of acute carbohydrate ingestion on anaerobic exercise performance. Journal of the International Society of Sports Nutrition,13, 40. https://doi.org/10.1186/s12970-016-0152-9

2. Burke, L. M., van Loon, L. J. C. & Hawley, J. A. (1985). Postexercise muscle glycogen resynthesis in humans. Journal of Applied Physiology, 122(5), 1055–1067. DOI: 10.1152/japplphysiol.00860.2016

3. Pascoe, D. D., Costill, D. L., Fink, W. J., Robergs, R. A. & Zachwieja, J. J. (1993). Glycogen resynthesis in skeletal muscle following resistive exercise. Medicine & Science in Sports & Exercise, 25(3), 349–354. PMID: 8455450

4. Pal, S. & Ellis, V. (2010). The acute effects of four protein meals on insulin, glucose, appetite and energy intake in lean men. British Journal of Nutrition, 104(8), 1241–1248. DOI: 10.1017/S0007114510001911

5. Koopman, R., Beelen, M., Stellingwerff, T., Pennings, B., Saris, W. H., Kies, A. K., Kuipers, H. & van Loon, L. J. (2007). Coingestion of carbohydrate with protein does not further augment postexercise muscle protein synthesis. American Journal of Physiology-Endocrinology and Metabolism, 293(3), E833–42. DOI: 10.1152/ajpendo.00135.2007

Chapter 14

1. Raynor, H. A. (2012). Can limiting dietary variety assist with reducing energy intake and weight loss? Physiology & Behavior, 106(3), 356–361. DOI: 10.1016/j.physbeh.2012.03.012

Chapter 16

1. Campos, G. E., Luecke, T. J., Wendeln, H. K., Toma, K., Hagerman, F. C., Murray, T. F., Ragg, K. E., Ratamess, N. A., Kraemer, W. J. & Staron, R. S. (2002, November). Muscular adaptations in response to three different resistance-training regimens: Specificity of repetition maximum training zones. European Journal of Applied Physiology, 88(1–2), 50–60. DOI: 10.1007/s00421-002-0681-6

2. Martorelli, S., Cadore, E. L., Izquierdo, M., Celes, R., Martorelli, A., Cleto, V. A., Alvarenga, J. G. & Bottaro, M. (2017, June 27). Strength training with repetitions to failure does not provide additional strength and muscle hypertrophy gains in young women. European Journal of Translational Myology, 27(2), 6339. DOI: 10.4081/ejtm.2017.6339

3. Ochi, E., Maruo, M., Tsuchiya, Y., Ishii, N., Miura, K. & Sasaki, K. (2018). Higher Training Frequency Is Important for Gaining Muscular Strength under Volume-Matched Training. Frontiers in Physiology, 9, 744. https://doi.org/10.3389/fphys.2018.00744

Chapter 17

1. Buresh, R., Berg, K. & French, J. (2009). The effect of resistive exercise rest interval on hormonal response, strength, and hypertrophy with training. Journal of Strength and Conditioning Research, 23(1), 62–71. DOI: 10.1519/JSC.0b013e318185f14a

2. Barroso, R., Silva-Batista, C., Tricoli, V., Roschel, H. & Ugrinowitsch, C. (2013). The effects of different intensities and durations of the general warm-up on leg press 1RM. Journal of Strength and Conditioning Research, 27(4), 1009–1013. https://doi.org/10.1519/JSC.0b013e3182606cd9

3. Behm, D. G. & Chaouachi, A. (2011). A review of the acute effects of static and dynamic stretching on performance. European Journal of Applied Physiology 111, 2633–2651. https://doi.org/10.1007/s00421-011-1879-2

Chapter 18

1. Spennewyn, K. C. (2008). Strength outcomes in fixed versus free-form resistance equipment. Journal of Strength and Conditioning Research, 22(1), 75–81. https://doi.org/10.1519/JSC.0b013e31815ef5e7

2. Goncalves, A., Gentil, P., Steele, J., Giessing, J., Paoli, A. & Fisher, J. P. (2019). Comparison of single- and multi-joint lower body resistance training upon strength increases in recreationally active males and females: A within-participant unilateral training study. European Journal of Translational Myology, 29(1), 8052. https://doi.org/10.4081/ejtm.2019.8052

3. McMahon, G. E., Onambélé-Pearson, G. L., Morse, C. I., Burden, A. M. & Winwood, K. (2013). How Deep Should You Squat to Maximise a Holistic Training Response? Electromyographic, Energetic, Cardiovascular, Hypertrophic and Mechanical Evidence. In (Ed.), Electrodiagnosis in New Frontiers of Clinical Research. IntechOpen. https://doi.org/10.5772/56386

4. Hilliard-Robertson, P. C., Schneider, S. M., Bishop, S. L. & Guilliams, M. E. (2003). Strength gains following different combined concentric and eccentric exercise regimens. Aviation, Space, and Environmental Medicine, 74(4), 342–347.

Chapter 19

1. Nunes, J. P., Grgic, J., Cunha, P. M., Ribeiro, A. S., Schoenfeld, B. J., de Salles, B. F. & Cyrino, E. S. (2020). What influence does resistance exercise order have on muscular strength gains and muscle hypertrophy? A systematic review and meta-analysis. European Journal of Sport Science, 21(2), 149–157. DOI: 10.1080/17461391.2020.1733672

Chapter 22

1. Björntorp, P. (1997). Hormonal control of regional fat distribution. Human Reproduction (Oxford, England), 12 Suppl 1, 21–25. https://doi.org/10.1093/humrep/12.suppl_1.21
2. Bartholomew, J. B., Stults-Kolehmainen, M. A., Elrod, C. C. & Todd, J. S. (2008). Strength gains after resistance training: The effect of stressful, negative life events. Journal of Strength and Conditioning Research, 22(4), 1215–1221. https://doi.org/10.1519/JSC.0b013e318173d0bf
3. Saner, N. J., Lee, M. J.-C., Pitchford, N. W., Kuang, J., Roach, G. D., Garnham, A., Stokes, T., Phillips, S. M., Bishop, D. J. & Bartlett, J. D. (2020). The effect of sleep restriction, with or without high-intensity interval exercise, on myofibrillar protein synthesis in healthy young men. Journal of Physiology, 598: 1523–1536. https://doi.org/10.1113/JP278828
4. Leproult, R. & Van Cauter, E. (2011). Effect of 1 week of sleep restriction on testosterone levels in young healthy men. JAMA, 305(21), 2173–2174. https://doi.org/10.1001/jama.2011.710
5. Leproult, R., Copinschi, G., Buxton, O. & Van Cauter, E. (1997). Sleep loss results in an elevation of cortisol levels the next evening. Sleep, 20(10), 865–870.
6. Donga, E., van Dijk, M., van Dijk, J. G., Biermasz, N. R., Lammers, G. J., van Kralingen, K. W., Corssmit, E. P. & Romijn, J. A. (2010). A single night of partial sleep deprivation induces insulin resistance in multiple metabolic pathways in healthy subjects. Journal of Clinical Endocrinology and Metabolism, 95(6), 2963–2968. https://doi.org/10.1210/jc.2009-2430
7. Buxton, O. M., Cain, S. W., O'Connor, S. P., Porter, J. H., Duffy, J. F., Wang, W., Czeisler, C. A. & Shea, S. A. (2012). Adverse metabolic consequences in humans of prolonged sleep restriction combined with circadian disruption. Science Translational Medicine, 4(129), 129ra43. https://doi.org/10.1126/scitranslmed.3003200
8. Bosy-Westphal, A., Hinrichs, S., Jauch-Chara, K., Hitze, B., Later, W., Wilms, B., Settler, U., Peters, A., Kiosz, D. & Müller, M. J. (2008). Influence of partial sleep deprivation on energy balance and insulin sensitivity in healthy women. Obesity Facts, 1(5), 266–273. DOI: 10.1159/000158874
9. Alhola, P. & Polo-Kantola, P. (2007). Sleep deprivation: Impact on cognitive performance. Neuropsychiatric Disease and Treatment, 3(5), 553–567.

10. Orzeł-Gryglewska, J. (2010). Consequences of sleep deprivation. International Journal of Occupational Medicine and Environmental Health, 23(1), 95–114. https://doi.org/10.2478/v10001-010-0004-9

11. Facer-Childs, E. R., Middleton, B., Skene, D. J. & Bagshaw, A. P. (2019). Resetting the late timing of 'night owls' has a positive impact on mental health and performance. Sleep Medicine, 60, 236–247. https://doi.org/10.1016/j.sleep.2019.05.001

12. Larsen, S. C. & Heitmann, B. L. (2019). More Frequent Intake of Regular Meals and Less Frequent Snacking Are Weakly Associated with Lower Long-Term Gains in Body Mass Index and Fat Mass in Middle-Aged Men and Women. Journal of Nutrition, 149(5), 824–830. https://doi.org/10.1093/jn/nxy326

13. Thomas, E. A., Higgins, J., Bessesen, D. H., McNair, B. & Cornier, M. A. (2015). Usual breakfast eating habits affect response to breakfast skipping in overweight women. Obesity (Silver Spring, Md.), 23(4), 750–759. https://doi.org/10.1002/oby.21049

14. Farshchi, H. R., Taylor, M. A. & Macdonald, I. A. (2004). Decreased thermic effect of food after an irregular compared with a regular meal pattern in healthy lean women. International Journal of Obesity and Related Metabolic Disorders: Journal of the International Association for the Study of Obesity, 28(5), 653–660. https://doi.org/10.1038/sj.ijo.0802616

15. Guinter, M. A., Park, Y. M., Steck, S. E. & Sandler, D. P. (2020). Day-to-day regularity in breakfast consumption is associated with weight status in a prospective cohort of women. International Journal of Obesity (2005), 44(1), 186–194. https://doi.org/10.1038/s41366-019-0356-6

Chapter 32

1.   Trecroci, A., Porcelli, S., Perri, E., Pedrali, M., Rasica, L., Alberti, G., Longo, S. & Iaia, F. M. (2020). Effects of different training interventions on the recovery of physical and neuromuscular performance after a soccer match. Journal of Strength and Conditioning Research, 34(8), 2189–2196. DOI: 10.1519/jsc.0000000000003269

Chapter 35

1.   Strasser, B., Spreitzer, A. & Haber, P. (2007). Fat loss depends on energy deficit only, independently of the method for weight loss. Annals of Nutrition & Metabolism, 51(5), 428–432. https://doi.org/10.1159/000111162

2.   Wilson, J. M., Marin, P. J., Rhea, M. R., Wilson, S. M., Loenneke, J. P. & Anderson, J. C. (2012). Concurrent training. Journal of Strength and Conditioning Research, 26(8), 2293–2307. DOI: 10.1519/jsc.0b013e31823a3e2d

3.   Jones, T. W., Howatson, G., Russell, M. & French, D. N. (2013). Performance and neuromuscular adaptations following differing ratios of concurrent strength and endurance training. Journal of Strength and Conditioning Research, 27(12), 3342–3351. DOI: 10.1519/jsc.0b013e3181b2cf39

4. Wilson, J. M., Marin, P. J., Rhea, M. R., Wilson, S. M., Loenneke, J. P., & Anderson, J. C. (2012). Concurrent training. Journal of Strength and Conditioning Research, 26(8), 2293–2307. DOI: 10.1519/jsc.0b013e31823a3e2d

5. Panissa, V. L. G., Fukuda, D. H., Staibano, V., Marques, M. & Franchini, E. (2020). Magnitude and duration of excess of post-exercise oxygen consumption between high-intensity interval and moderate-intensity continuous exercise: A systematic review. Obesity Reviews, 22(1). DOI: 10.1111/obr.13099

6. Panissa, V. L. G., Fukuda, D. H., Staibano, V., Marques, M., & Franchini, E. (2020). Magnitude and duration of excess of post-exercise oxygen consumption between high-intensity interval and moderate-intensity continuous exercise: A systematic review. Obesity Reviews, 22(1). DOI: 10.1111/obr.13099

7. de Souza, E. O., Tricoli, V., Aoki, M. S., Roschel, H., Brum, P. C., Bacurau, A. V., Silva-Batista, C., Wilson, J. M., Neves, M., Soares, A. G. & Ugrinowitsch, C. (2014). Effects of concurrent strength and endurance training on genes related to myostatin signaling pathway and muscle fiber responses. Journal of Strength and Conditioning Research, 28(11), 3215–3223. DOI: 10.1519/jsc.0000000000000525

8. Keating, S. E., Machan, E. A., O'Connor, H. T., Gerofi, J. A., Sainsbury, A., Caterson, I. D. & Johnson, N. A. (2014). Continuous exercise but not high intensity interval training improves fat distribution in overweight adults. Journal of Obesity, 1–12. DOI: 10.1155/2014/834865

9. Tremblay, A., Simoneau, J. A. & Bouchard, C. (1994). Impact of exercise intensity on body fatness and skeletal muscle metabolism. Metabolism, 43(7), 814–818. DOI: 10.1016/0026-0495(94)90259-3

Chapter 36

1. Fairfield, K. M. & Fletcher, R. H. (2002, June). Vitamins for chronic disease prevention in adults: Scientific review. Journal of the American Medical Association, 287(23), 3116–26. DOI: 10.1001/jama.287.23.3116

2. Albert, B. B., Derraik, J. G. B., Cameron-Smith, D., Hofman, P. L., Tumanov, S., Villas-Boas, S. G., Garg, M. L. & Cutfield, W. S. (2016). Erratum: Corrigendum: Fish oil supplements in New Zealand are highly oxidised and do not meet label content of n-3 PUFA. Scientific Reports, 6(1). DOI: 0.1038/srep35092

3. Duncan, M. J., Stanley, M., Parkhouse, N., Cook, K. & Smith, M. (2013). Acute caffeine ingestion enhances strength performance and reduces perceived exertion and muscle pain perception during resistance exercise. European Journal of Sport Science, 13(4), 392–399. DOI: 10.1080/17461391.2011.635811

4. Davis, J. & Green, J. M. (2009). Caffeine and anaerobic performance. Sports Medicine, 39(10), 813–832. DOI: 10.2165/11317770-000000000-00000

5. Ferreira, G., Felippe, L., Bertuzzi, R., Bishop, D., Ramos, I., De-Oliveira, F. & Lima-Silva, A. (2019). Does caffeine ingestion before a short-term sprint interval training promote body fat loss? Brazilian Journal of Medical and Biological Research, 52(12). DOI: 10.1590/1414-431x20199169

6. Wilk, M., Filip, A., Krzysztofik, M., Maszczyk, A. & Zajac, A. (2019). The acute effect of various doses of caffeine on power output and velocity during the bench press exercise among athletes habitually using caffeine. Nutrients, 11(7), 1465. DOI: 10.3390/nu11071465

7. Elliot, T. A., Cree, M. G., Sanford, A. P., Wolfe, R. R. & Tipton, K. D. (2006). Milk ingestion stimulates net muscle protein synthesis following resistance exercise. Medicine & Science in Sports & Exercise, 38(4), 667–674. DOI: 10.1249/01.mss.0000210190.64458.25

8. Elliot, T. A., Cree, M. G., Sanford, A. P., Wolfe, R. R., & Tipton, K. D. (2006). Milk ingestion stimulates net muscle protein synthesis following resistance exercise. Medicine & Science in Sports & Exercise, 38(4), 667–674. DOI: 10.1249/01.mss.0000210190.64458.25

9. Chan, A. H., D'Souza, R. F., Beals, J. W., Zeng, N., Prodhan, U., Fanning, A. C., Poppitt, S. D., Li, Z., Burd, N. A., Cameron-Smith, D. & Mitchell, C. J. (2019, September). The degree of aminoacidemia after dairy protein ingestion does not modulate the postexercise anabolic response in young men: A randomized controlled trial. Journal of Nutrition, 149(9), 1511–1522. DOI: 10.1093/jn/nxz099

10. Branch, J. D. (2003). Effect of creatine supplementation on body composition and performance: A meta-analysis. International Journal of Sport Nutrition and Exercise Metabolism, 13(2), 198–226. DOI: 10.1123/ijsnem.13.2.198

11. Trexler, E. T., Smith-Ryan, A. E., Stout, J. R., et al. (2015). International Society of Sports Nutrition Position Stand: Beta-Alanine. Journal of the International Society of Sports Nutrition, 12, 30. https://doi.org/10.1186/s12970-015-0090-y

12. Trexler, E. T., Smith-Ryan, A. E., Stout, J. R., et al. (2015). International Society of Sports Nutrition Position Stand: Beta-Alanine. Journal of the International Society of Sports Nutrition, 12, 30. https://doi.org/10.1186/s12970-015-0090-y

Printed in Great Britain
by Amazon

21445949R00167